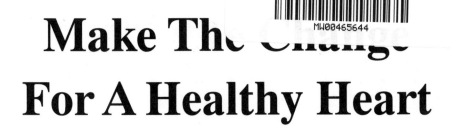

Make The Change
For A Healthy Heart

The Powerful, New, Commonsense Approach
to Preventing and Reversing Heart Disease

Frank Barry, M.D.

With Bridget Swinney, M.S., R.D.

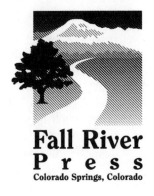

Fall River
P r e s s
Colorado Springs, Colorado

©1995 by Frank Barry and Bridget Swinney

Fall River Press
P.O Box 62578
Colorado Springs, CO 80962-2578
(719) 590-9464

Publisher's Cataloging in Publication
(Prepared by Quality Books, Inc.)

Barry, Frank J.
    Make the change for a healthy heart : the powerful, new, Commonsense approach to preventing and reversing heart disease / Frank Barry and Bridget Swinney. -- Colorado Springs, Colo. : Fall River Press, 1995.
    p.cm.
    Includes bibliographical references and index.
    ISBN 0–9632917–2-6

    1. Heart--Diseases--Prevention.   2. Cardiovascular system--Diseases-Prevention.   I. Swinney, Bridget, 1960- II. Title.

RC681.B37 1995   616.1'205
                                      QBI95-20361

            Library of Congress Catalog Card Number: 95-061084

Cover design and illustration:	Gortwood & Associates
Typesetting and graphic design:	Frank Blando
Cartoons:	Pat Steinholtz
Back cover photograph:	Wayne Valey
Inside photograph:	Tini Campbell
Printed by:	Publishers Press Inc.
Nutritional Analysis of recipes:	Nutritionist III™,
	N-Squared Computing, Salem Oregon

Praise for Make The Change For a Healthy Heart

"Finally--A heart-healthy book full of realistic, commonsense ideas."

Jacquie Craig, M.S., R.D., C.D.E.

"This book is a wonderful, practical guide to a healthy heart. I highly recommend it!"

Peggy Huddleston, Psychotherapist, author of *Prepare for Surgery, Heal Faster: A Guide of Mind-Body Techniques.*

"An easy, fast, information-packed read that covers not only making the necessary changes for a healthy heart, but is a pertinent and interesting compilation of facts that can benefit the reader in a myriad of ways."

Helen J. Ginsburg, author of *From The Heart; Overcoming The Mental and Physical Trauma of Open Heart Surgery* and Spokesperson, American Heart Association of Colorado

"Make the Change for a Healthy Heart" is the best organized, most thorough treatment of the subject that I have come across. Your book allows anyone wishing to minimize their risk factors to get a complete review of the subject in one book. It will certainly fill a niche that has sadly been left empty for too many years. I wish I would have had access to such a book for my patients years ago."

G. Scott Smith M.D., F. A.C.C.
Cardiologist

"Make the Change for a Healthy Heart is a valuable addition for preventing, treatment and even reversing coronary artery disease through appropriate dieting, stress management and exercise. It provides the patient an opportunity to take charge and play a very active role in prevention and reversal of coronary artery disease, the number one killer."

Mark V. Barrow, M.D., Ph.D.
Gainesville Cardiology and Medical Center

Acknowledgments

As a first time author, I had no idea how difficult this project would turn out to be. I hope you the reader will gain from perusing this book.

I want to thank my family, Mary, Colleen, and Megan for putting up with my hours in front of the computer. Also to Bridget Swinney for help in the dietary arena, and as a valued contributor.

I owe a debt of gratitude to my friend and author Zoltan Malocsay, for the invaluable assistance he provided. Susan Hyne spent many hours editing and her suggestions were right on the mark. G. Scott Smith, cardiologist extraordinaire, has been supportive through the process and added his expertise to the revisions. I am eternally grateful.

The staff of the Preventive Health Institute, including Craig Engle L.C.S.W., Laurin McCrary M.S. have lent their expertise and enthusiasm.

My extended family, including "Uncle Dave" Howes and Aunt Dorothy Zimmerman have taught me more on a practical level than words can say.

As a medical professional, I wish to pay homage to the giants in the field: the real pioneer Nathan Pritikin and to Kenneth Cooper, M.D.; John McDougall, M.D.; Dean Ornish M.D.

A private word to all my patients who taught me the practical aspects of their lives, and by doing so, brightened my life immeasurable. Thank you all for sharing such intimacy with your physician.

My only wish is that you could have known my father as I did. He was an exceptional man.

Frank Barry, M.D.
May 1, 1995
Colorado Springs, Colorado

I wish to first thank my husband, Frank and my sons Nicolas and Robert for their patience while I spent many hours at the computer and made many messes in the kitchen. And to my sisters, Judy and Colleen, my Dad and Nicole for all their support.

I'd like to thank Frank Barry for getting me involved in the Preventive Health Institute--who would have known that it would lead to a book! Also, for giving my husband the knowledge he needed about heart disease to learn that he did have a choice.

I'd also like to thank all my friends and co-workers for their support especially Wayne Valey, Kathy Glaaser R.D., Kathy Fraser, Jacquie Craig R.D., Ann Snyder R.D. from the Gladstone Institute, and Mary Peet R.D.

And for help in tasting products and testing recipes: Kathy Fraser, Julie Branscomb, Debbie Russell, Lori Hannah R.D. Norma Robinson R.D., Janet Boyd, and Sheryl Stampher R.D., Ceacy Thatcher, Nancy Oshner, Todd Rowader R.N., Wendy Gregor R.D., Dan Mayotte, Carol Williams and Tina Fulton. Thanks to Ceacy Thatcher, Patty Magliato, Norma Robinson R.D., and Shirley Lippincott R.D. for the use of their recipes. Kudos to Cecile Gort for wonderful cover art and helpful advice!

Thanks to my colleagues at Memorial Hospital and the Spring 1995 Behavior Modification Weight Loss Classes at Memorial Hospital for help in tasting fat-free products and recipes.

Bridget Swinney, M.S., R.D.

<u>Important!</u>

Make the Change for a Healthy Heart is a program of life-style changes that can reverse and prevent heart disease. It is not meant to take the place of medical advice from your personal physician. You should always contact your physician before starting a program of diet or exercise. The Make the Change Meal Plan is not meant for people with special nutrient needs such as pregnant women or children. For further dietary advice for special needs, seek the advice of a registered dietitian or your physician.

About the Authors

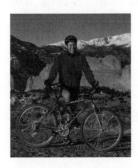

Frank Barry, MD practices family medicine and sports medicine in Colorado. Born in Jersey City, New Jersey, he moved to Colorado fifteen years ago to take a residency in Family Medicine at the University of Colorado Health Sciences Center in Denver. He has always been interested in the whole person, not just their disease.

He received both his Bachelor of Science degree in psychology and his MD degree from Georgetown University. Disease prevention became an avocation after several years in practice. Family events also played a role. Sports medicine and exercise science helped in triathlons, century bike rides and outdoor sports to which he aspires.

He lives the lifestyle he teaches at the Preventive Health Institute. His wife, an RN with a Master's Degree in Sports Science, and their two girls frequently bike, camp and play soccer together. Doctor Barry is the President of the El Paso County Medical Society. He lives and works in beautiful Colorado Springs, Colorado.

Contributing author Bridget Swinney is a registered dietitian with a Master's Degree in Nutrition. She is author of *Eating Expectantly; The Essential Eating Guide and Cookbook for Pregnancy,* which was chosen as one of the Ten Best Parenting Books of 1993 by *Child Magazine.* She works as an outpatient dietitian and consultant in Colorado Springs.

PREVENTIVE HEALTH INSTITUTE

On the day of my college graduation I was awakened by a call from my parents' hotel. My father had just died of a sudden heart attack!

He was only 53.

Stunned, devastated, I remember wondering if this is all that life is about: Work hard, get plenty of "standard medical care" and drop dead before you can see your child graduate. To lots of people, that's all there is. Millions die early, suddenly, needlessly. That was my introduction to heart disease, America's number one killer.

I went on to medical school at Georgetown, thinking that life should be better than what my father suffered--longer than that, richer, fuller, with time to enjoy family and accomplishments. But I was scared because a family history of heart disease is a major risk factor. Now the Grim Reaper had his finger at me, whispering "Next?"

As it turned out, my aunt was next.

When my aunt Dorothy had a heart attack, I was immersed in the usual medical training. Don't "blame" patients for their illness. Don't expect a measure of personal responsibility from people for their health. Drugs are the first line of defense. Surgery is the ultimate defense. If these don't work, write the patient off with the deadly dismissal "there's nothing else we can do."

But Aunt Dorothy wouldn't stand for that. She had been the picture of health! So when I learned that her cholesterol level was over 300, I was shocked. Then she started to have allergic reactions to all the cholesterol-lowering drugs, and I got frightened. What could I do to help? Immediately I thought of surgery, but she wanted to explore other possibilities. Yes, I had heard of Nathan Pritikin, but wasn't he a kook from California?

Dorothy's remarkable recovery from heart disease on a program of lowfat eating and exercise not only piqued my interest, it made me eternally thankful! At last, I saw something that worked!

I researched the work of Kenneth Cooper, M.D., inventor of the "aerobics" concept. His continuing work has been accepted and embraced by the sports medicine community, if not the heart disease community. My brother-in-law introduced me to the work of John McDougall, M.D. and the concept that disease could be cured by proper nutrition. Anne Frahm's *A Cancer Battle Plan* introduced me to the term "SAD," for Standard American Diet. Could all the favorite American foods like burgers, fries, and shakes which I had enjoyed my whole life be causing the diseases which plague modern Americans? The evidence was mounting.

As I continued my study of heart disease and prevention, I became interested in cholesterol and its metabolism. Imagine my surprise when, at a conference, I learned that an integrated approach of diet, exercise, and stress reduction advocated by Dean Ornish, M.D., had actually **reversed** heart disease! I considered this a world-class scientific achievement! No longer would doctors "plug the hole" in the proverbial dike. We could actually reverse the number one killer!

Nevertheless, the general medical community remains uncomfortable about implementing these advances. And there are no internationally known pharmaceutical companies willing to fund further research on the beneficial effects of a lowfat diet on heart disease and cancer. The standard medical protocols remain "usual and customary care." If Americans don't take control of their own care, then "usual and customary" is all they're going to get.

THE PURPOSE OF THIS BOOK

It was frustration--even desperation--that urged me to found the Preventive Health Institute. I wanted to put all these new tools to work!

The Preventive Health Institute is a team of professionals from the fields of exercise physiology, mental health, nutrition, and medicine who work together to teach people- victims of heart disease and hardening of the arteries- to take back control of their lives. Based in Colorado Springs, Colorado, away from academic medical centers, the Institute has been successful in helping ordinary people rather than "subjects" in a research program. This highly personal approach made us concentrate on **down-to-earth** interventions to change the health and lives of working people.

We have found out what other programs haven't: why most prevention / reversal programs fail. As it turns out, the answer is as clear as the nose on your face.

People go for the small "easy" changes at first. When a small, hard-to-measure benefit occurs, most just give up with a "what's the use?" They don't feel better, they just feel deprived. "Wow, my cholesterol dropped 5 points--Big deal."

The secret: big changes, big benefits. All at once. After a week or two, when you don't need to look for benefits with a magnifying glass because you already feel them, you'll be happy. The improvements will keep you coming back for more.

So what follows is a truly **practical** program to prevent and reverse heart and vascular disease for those willing to make the changes. This program actually works to help those at most risk. By good fortune, it is an excellent information source for worried spouses and loved ones. Even more, the program demonstrates a lifestyle that can benefit everyone who is willing to make the change to a better life.

But I know what you're thinking; I know what you fear.

You don't want to live like a hamster, caged by your disease, forced to eat a hamster's diet and exercise endlessly on a hamster's treadmill, just to save your miserable life.

That's no life for a human being. I agree.

And that's why you've opened the right book! This is not a program of deprivation and hardship; this is a program of abundance and fun. Once you MAKE THE CHANGE, *you can rid yourself of your disease and free yourself from its cage. At last, you'll find yourself in a world that is a grand buffet of delicious and exciting foods, an unfolding abundance of different eating pleasures.* You can live a wonderful life with less stress and more fun! You can become more active, stronger, better able to enjoy each new day. With some practical help- and an open mind- you can literally eat, drink, and be merry, live to enjoy your family and your accomplishments as my father never did.

Sound too good to be true? You'll earn the results, believe me! It'll take some doing, some work, some close attention because this is applied science, not magic. But we call this a **practical** guide because you really can do it, and it really does work. If you MAKE THE CHANGE, you can be the living proof just like the others who've tried.

My prescription is: **MAKE THE CHANGE!**

CHAPTER 1

TWENTY FIRST CENTURY MEDICINE

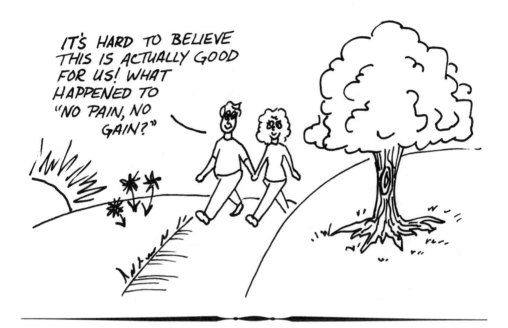

"To boldly go where no man has gone before."

Star Trek

Imagine a loved one experiencing chest pains. His doctor thinks it's due to blockage of a heart artery. He is told to take medication (a beta blocker and nitroglycerine). Dutifully following advice, he finds he has headaches and feels tired as side effects. He can no longer take his daily walk because of fatigue.

When he returns to the doctor, a check on his cholesterol shows it is rising. The chest discomfort, although better, is still present. He is referred to a cardiologist.

The cardiologist is a caring, cautious man. After reviewing the results of a treadmill test, which has several minor abnormalities, he recommends cardiac catheterization. The Operative Permit states, "I will cut a small hole in your artery, and push a catheter through it into your heart. Then, after injecting dye into the catheter, I will take a series of pictures. These will show any blockage. Side effects are minimal, but include bleeding, infection, damage to the artery, and cardiac arrest."

The test is scheduled the next day. Although apprehensive, the patient sails through without complications. However, when reviewing the results, the cardiologist notes blockages of 75% in the right coronary artery, and 30-40% in the left anterior descending and left circumflex arteries. (These are the 3 largest, most important sources of nourishment to the heart.) In his conference with the patient, he dismisses the left artery blockages as "minimal." The right artery must, however, have immediate angioplasty to "avoid a heart attack." The patient, frightened, agrees and has an angioplasty the next day. The balloon is blown up, crushing the plaque, partially dilating the artery.

Six months later, on-and-off chest pain returns. The patient immediately sees the cardiologist, who orders immediate catheterization. The site of the angioplasty is, unfortunately, completely blocked. In addition, the left artery blockages look "ratty" or irregular. In conference with the patient, the cardiologist recommends immediate bypass surgery, and sends in the surgeon.

The surgeon, after agreeing with the cardiologist, says there is time in his schedule tomorrow. Otherwise, "you might have to wait till next week, and I don't know what might happen in the meantime."

The patient, shivering, feeling ill and terrified, agrees. He signs the permit, which states, "After putting you to sleep, we use a small saw to cut your sternum (breastbone). Your heart is then stopped. Your circulation is controlled by machine pump. Veins from your leg are used to bypass the blocked arteries. Your heart is then re-started. Possible side effects are infection, bleeding, pneumonia, heart attack, stroke, and death."

At surgery the next day, the surgeon finds a scar on the heart, indicative of a heart attack from the right artery blockage. He is able to bypass the right and both left arteries. The patient recovers and is ready to go home.

On the day of hospital discharge, the surgeon says "the operation was a complete success. I was able to bypass the blockages. Except for the little scar I found, your heart is working well. Go home, be careful, eat right, exercise, reduce stress, and enjoy yourself. Any questions?"

As the patient opens his mouth to ask "but doctor, how long will my surgery last?," the surgeon is out the door. "See you in two weeks in the office. I have another emergency surgery to perform."

The patient leaves feeling perplexed. "Am I cured? Then why do I have to be careful? And just what does 'eat right' mean, anyhow? And how do I enjoy myself if I can't enjoy myself?"

...NOW, A PEEK INTO THE FUTURE...

The patient's granddaughter is watching a hologram from her dear, departed grandad:

How fortunate you are, Sarah. From your early years in junior high school when you were 8, through college at age 14, you have been exposed to the concepts of 21st century medicine. And now you will be a doctor! I am very proud and also more than a little relieved.

Today, heart disease and hardening of the arteries is not the problem it once was. Instead of waiting for disease to happen, doctors believe that "an ounce of prevention is worth a pound of cure." They teach everyone exactly how and why they can prevent the major killers. They have refined "pleasurable" risk reduction to a science. Let me tell you how things have changed since I had my heart attack.

After meat advertising was banned, people realized they had many choices in food and other aspects of their life-style, and felt less pressure to make bad health choices. And when these choices led not only to heart health, but less cancer and greater happiness, the movement grew. Research proved the power of good mental attitude. "Believing is seeing," (using the power of your will to make positive change--rather than seeing is believing) and positive attitude became powerful therapeutic tools of medicine.

Now, of course, everyone exercises, even those with disease. We know exercise helps rather than hurts a damaged heart.

The pursuit of personal satisfaction, after setting clearly defined goals, became the "vaccine" of 2010. As more people were **expected** to take personal responsibility for their health, more actually did so. With the power of food to prevent disease, instead of cause it, and the vaccine of happiness, coupled with education on good and bad choices, the world is a better place to live. Since women are now treated equally to men in medicine, in professional opportunity and in the therapy of disease, you, Sarah, can practice the 21st century specialty, the specialty of practical proven prevention. HERE'S TO YOUR HEART, YOUR HEALTH, AND YOUR HAPPINESS. Prevent heart disease so your patients won't have to reverse it.

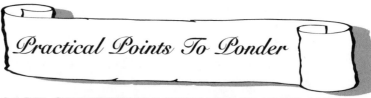

Practical Points To Ponder

21ST CENTURY MEDICINE TODAY

The Preventive Health Institute practices 21st century medicine. I will present detailed descriptions of pleasurable, concise, and practical guidelines on food and its power to heal, stress reduction and its therapeutic effects, and exercise.

- ♥ All the people who come to the Preventive Health Institute have one thing in common. They have heart disease (hardening of the arteries). They have been helped by 21st century medicine.

- ♥ Those concerned with **preventing** heart disease or stroke can also benefit.

- ♥ Anyone planning for a healthy, long, happy retirement would be well advised to follow the Pleasurable Risk Reduction Plan. It lets you enjoy the fruit of your labor, alongside your family.

- ♥ Either learn to live with your disease, or learn to get rid of the disease!
- ♥ Get rid of side effects that make you feel ill.

PLEASURABLE RISK REDUCTION

From a concept by David S. Sobel (used with permission from Robert Ornstein and David Sobel: Healthy Pleasures. New York: Addison-Wesley, 1989). (Reference 1 and reference 2)

The following are powerful predictors of future cardiac health. They also can help you "feel like" making the change:

- ♥ Happiness and lack of depression
- ♥ Marital satisfaction
- ♥ Higher education level
- ♥ Owning a pet
- ♥ Taking a nap or slowing down on the job
- ♥ Having 1 or 2 drinks of alcohol a day (only if you already drink!)
- ♥ Gentle, pleasurable physical activity most every day
- ♥ Based on a close look at your personal goals, make appropriate health-enhancing choices about your food, your job, your family and your happiness

Make the change! Get rid of your disease.

THE PROOF

I will briefly review the scientific studies showing the benefits of 21st century medicine in reversing heart disease. If you or your doctor have questions, look up the scientific references. It is very important to have a rational, reasonable plan before you embark on the changes outlined in this book. Convince yourself that this plan will work for you. (See also suggested reading, page 325)

DIET AND EXERCISE

♥ Lifestyle Heart Trial. Proves that people with hardening of the arteries can reverse the disease without medicine or surgery. Changes included a 10% lowfat vegetarian diet, smoking cessation, comprehensive stress management, and exercise.

Of interest, the control group got worse. They stayed on the American Heart Association's Step 2 diet (27% fat). (Reference 3)

♥ St. Thomas Atheroma Regression Study. One arm of this study consisted of a 27% lowfat diet, weight loss to ideal body weight, and daily exercise. Regression of heart disease was seen in 38% of this group. Another part of this study used drugs and was also successful. (Reference 4)

DRUGS, DIET AND EXERCISE

♥ Coronary Drug Project. Proved that nicotinic acid or niacin reduced recurrent heart attacks, 8.9% vs. 12.2% after 6 years. Also, after 10 years, all-cause death was reduced, 58.2% vs. 52%. (Reference 5)

- ♥ Pravastatin Multi-National Study Group for Cardiac Risk Patients. Proved that pravastatin reduced the risk of serious cardiovascular events, 0.2% vs. 2.4%, after 6 months (Reference 6)

- ♥ Familial Atherosclerosis Treatment Study. Proved that two sets of drugs (lovastatin and colestipol, and niacin and colestipol), both lowered cholesterol and caused regression (32% for lovastatin and 39% for niacin groups). (Reference 7)

- ♥ Cholesterol Lowering Atherosclerosis Study. Proved that after bypass surgery, a lowfat diet, colestipol and niacin caused regression in 18% after 4 years, vs. 6.4% of controls. (Reference 8)

- ♥ Scandinavian Simvastatin Survival Study. Proved that a cholesterol-lowering drug reduced, in 5.4 years, the overall risk of death by 30%. Also decreased the risk of coronary death by 42%. All participants had previous heart disease. (Reference 9)

  Expert physicians, commenting on this study, feel it will enable doctors to treat heart disease differently, with less surgery and angioplasty.

Greater benefits are gained from greater lowering of the LDL cholesterol, the "bad" cholesterol. How low? It is Dr. William Castelli's opinion (the director of the landmark Framingham heart study), that an LDL cholesterol of 150 or less is protective of heart attack in almost all circumstances!

The benefits of 21st century medicine overall consist of reduction in chest pain, heart attack, and stroke (the benefits even extend to decrease in cancer). Even those without regression who were successful in reducing LDL cholesterol benefited! The magnitude was in some studies 70 - 80% reduction in bad outcomes compared to the control group!

CHAPTER 2

THE PROBLEM WITH HEART DISEASE

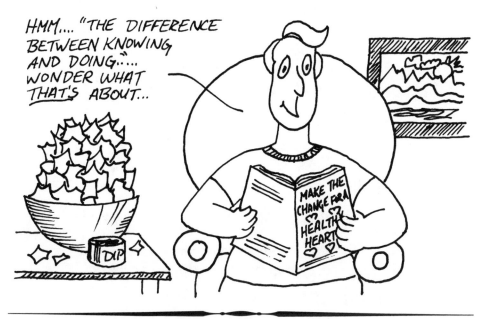

> *"Live Sensibly - Among 1000 people, only one dies a natural death, the rest succumb to irrational modes of living."*

Maimonides
12th century physician

A buddy of mine, retired from the insurance business, told me what the problem with heart disease was. "I sold retirement plans for years. Save a little now, get back a lot when you need it. Money to travel, live on, enjoy the fruits of a life's work. But heart disease is like inflation. It cheapens everything. Now that I'm ready, it's worth less than when I started. I'm out of time. My heart is giving up on me!"

As she died that night in the Intensive Care Unit, husband at her side, all the retirement planning in the world didn't change her family's grief. For her, it didn't matter. Life was over.

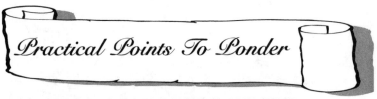

Practical Points To Ponder

SIGNS OF REVERSING HEART DISEASE

You know you are starting to reverse heart disease when:

- ♥ You feel better.
- ♥ You lose weight.
- ♥ Your cholesterol drops.
- ♥ Your physical endurance increases.
- ♥ Your chest pain diminishes, then vanishes.

INTRODUCTION

There is a difference between knowing and doing. Knowledge makes for interesting research and reading.

However, when human lives are at stake, knowing is not enough.

The **practical** aspects of our program are designed to enhance the doing. Research proves this program works in a way not possible with drugs or surgery. Now, take control of your heart, your health, and your happiness. And enjoy it!

This is 21st century medicine, available now. Many physicians think people are **too dumb or too disinterested** to learn how to help themselves. However, there is a large and growing movement of consumerism in the health field. People can and do make the decision to **help themselves**.

Most of us today seek safety and control. Safety from crime, poverty, and disease. Control over our lives. Recent medical research has proven that heart disease can be prevented and even reversed! What does this mean? The hardening of the arteries which caused you to have angioplasty, or bypass surgery, or a heart attack, can be opened up again. You can also learn the motivation to remain healthy in every way-- physically, mentally and emotionally. You can achieve both safety and control.

Food for Thought:

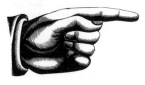

You can gain the power of food, exercise, stress reduction and group support. Lack of side effects. Freedom from the expense, pain and loss of control of standard medical therapy. Proven results. 21st century medicine, available now. Make the change!

How can this program help you? It definitely has the potential to improve your physical health. In addition, it can help you enjoy your life more fully, opening up new possibilities. Cancer prevention is likewise available. If these changes translate into **longevity** and **vigor**, so much the better. Even if they do not, however, the rest of your life can be lived to the fullest, enjoying all the pleasures life has to offer.

Many people spend their time feeling **powerless** about health and emotional well-being, **trapped** by inertia and depression, isolated from deep human contact.They make it a habit to give away their power. Others "learn" maladaptive behavior patterns which have outgrown their usefulness. Some feel unable to communicate, misunderstood. These behaviors can be changed; the power to see and enjoy each day to the fullest can be learned again (or for some, for the first time). This leads to vastly increased productivity, creativity, energy, vigor and satisfaction.

The knowledge conveyed in this program, coupled with a healthy dose of "believing is seeing," can lead to empowerment. Believe first, and it will happen. Wait to see it first, and it will never happen. The willpower and motivation to change comes from **regaining control** of your life. And once that step is accomplished, there is no limit to the positive benefits that take place.

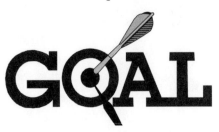

Doctors used to believe that "aging" was inevitable. The more birthdays, the greater the inevitable decline in function: sexually, in daily vigor, and especially in heart strength. **This is not true!** Most of what we call "aging" is disuse (mental and physical), despair, and the ravages of an excessive lifestyle. That these factors can be reversed has now been medically proven (Reference 3). What we will convey, in a practical manner, is the **"how" to accomplish your goal.**

You may likewise be interested in remaining "independent." For many, this means staying out of a nursing home, for others, travelling the world! Whatever it means to you, it may very well be your primary concern. You enhance your chance for an independent lifestyle with the knowledge gained in our program and this book.

One of my favorite people is Florence. She used to be sick. But something happened, inside her head. She decided to get well... And she did! Years ago, she embarked on her journey, did her own research. Exercise, eating right, improved attitude. She got rid of her problems instead of living with them.

Today, at 80, Florence has slowed down some. But she still takes her daily walk, and loves to regale me with stories. Although her old friends have passed away, she makes plenty of new ones. What a sharp mind. What a remarkable woman!

Please, help us help you. Start with an open mind. It's imperative to question, but leave a little skepticism behind. Try the "believing is seeing" attitude on for size. You may find that as you feel better, you will like the way it fits the new you.

CARDIOVASCULAR DISEASE STATES

I'll never forget an old veteran named Harry. A diabetic, he was one of my first patients at the Veterans Administration Hospital.

Harry was an engaging fellow, always smiling and ready with a joke. We got to see each other quite a few times during my medical training. Because of his diabetes and smoking, Harry had severe hardening of the arteries. This first affected his legs, and the pain of claudication (pain with activity, relief at rest) slowed him down.

But not his wit! It was always a pleasure to care for Harry. Through medical control of the diabetes, after angioplasty on the leg arteries, and during his aorto-femoral bypass surgery, the stories, the humor endured.

When the diabetes affected his vision, however, Harry seemed to fade. He was still pleasant, and always had a kind word for his doctors. But he was not the same.

The last year of his life was not a happy one for Harry. George, his son, was to graduate from high school. Angina, blindness, and recurring leg ulcers made life painful to bear. But Harry had a goal--to attend his son's graduation. When the heart attack came, we all thought he would never make it out of the hospital, much less to the graduation. Kidney failure, brought on by the fluid pills, made the situation worse.

The will to survive is strong. And Harry had a will. He pulled through, with a little help from kidney dialysis, and went home. Weakened, almost blind, he did survive to attend his son's graduation, and died soon after.

His son was kind enough to let know that Harry appreciated all the care. It was bittersweet, feeling his kindness while seeing him suffer and deteriorate.

By far, the largest cause of preventable disease and death is cardiovascular disease. This includes clogging of the arteries all over the body. In the brain and neck (carotid artery), this can lead to stroke, memory loss, dementia, loss of independence. This is termed "multi-infarct dementia."

In the legs, it causes claudication (pain with activity, relief at rest) and gangrene (death of the toes and feet). In the kidneys, failure leads to dialysis.

And in the heart, the clogging and eventual clotting can cause angina or chest pain, heart failure, heart attack (myocardial infarction) and even sudden death. These cause over a million deaths yearly. About half the people with heart attacks each year never make it to a hospital, never get the benefits of the "clot busting" drugs, but simply die suddenly. These deaths number over 450,000 yearly. Lumped together, this process of clogging and failure of the arteries is called atherosclerosis. (Figure 1)

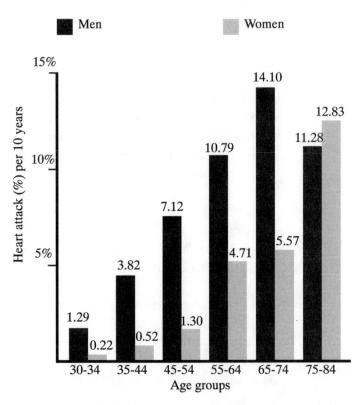

Figure 1. Incidence of myocardial infarction changes with sex and age. From the Framingham study of 5127 people (Reference 10)

DOCTOR, HOW LONG WILL MY SURGERY LAST?

Therapy of atherosclerosis traditionally falls into two categories: medicines and surgery. The many medicines can give benefit to some, but the side effects may, and often do, outweigh the limited improvement (More on drugs in chapter 12).

Surgery falls into two types, angioplasty and **coronary artery bypass grafting** (CABG).

Angioplasty sounds great! Just push a balloon catheter through the artery until it crosses the blockage, blow it up, and blow the blockage away! Unfortunately, up to 50% of the blockages are back after only six months. In addition, the fracturing of the artery that occurs with each angioplasty can lead to bleeding and emergency surgery. Further, a clot often forms, causing the newly opened artery to have no blood flow due to the clot, rather than the atherosclerosis. Incredibly, research in the prestigious *New England Journal of Medicine (NEJM)* found that angioplasty may be overutilized by at least 50%! (Reference 10 and reference 11) That is, at least one out of every two procedures is unnecessary! Over 300,000 angioplasties a year are performed in the USA at a cost of $15,000 to $20,000 each.

CABG surgery is at least as well known. There is good evidence that enhanced **survival** occurs in selected groups (left main artery blockage, three vessel coronary artery disease, reduced left ventricle function, and two vessel coronary disease when the LAD artery is involved). (Figure 2) However, most CABG surgery is done because of problems other than those listed above. Frequently, relief of chest pain is the goal. Research in the *New England Journal of Medicine* states that CABG is also overused one out of two times! It is performed about 260,000 times a year, at a cost of $40,000 to $50,000 a surgery. Seventy percent of vein grafts are occluded at 10 years! It caused heart attack in 8% as a direct result of the surgery! (Reference 11) Isn't there a better way?

Coronary Artery

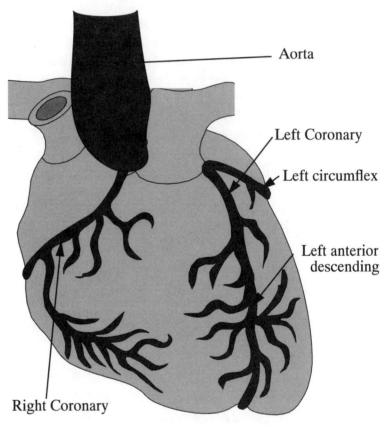

Aorta

Left Coronary

Left circumflex

Left anterior
descending

Right Coronary

Figure 2.

RISK FACTORS

IF THIS SECTION IS TOO TECHNICAL FOR YOUR
PLEASURE, TURN TO "PRACTICAL POINTS TO
PONDER", WHICH FOLLOWS AT THE END OF THIS
CHAPTER.

How is hardening of the arteries preventable and reversible? Doctors know that cardiovascular disease is caused by various **risk factors**. Reduce these and things improve. For you, this translates into less disease and disability, and prevents early death. Change these risk factors radically, and you can reverse damage already done. Let's get started.

CHOLESTEROL

I want to let you in on genetics. Many have given up the idea of changing their cholesterol levels. Stu was one of them. His father died at age 36. When Stu came to see me, he was 36 years old. It's true, he had a genetic form of high cholesterol. With a value of 350, he knew he had problems coming, but fast!

What he didn't realize is the power of 21st century medicine to reduce risk. We worked hard on a program of exercise, lowfat eating, and 40 mg. a day of a powerful cholesterol drug called simvistatin. One month later, a much happier Stu found his cholesterol to be 225. Not perfect, but a heck of a lot better.

"I feel an early death, like my father's, is not inevitable now. I have a lot to live for, and now I see a way to enjoy life. The monkey is off my back!" Stu continues to lead a healthy life. He has even lowered his cholesterol below 200. And he doesn't fear death on a day-to-day basis anymore!

DIETARY FAT = CHOLESTEROL. Let me explain. The body needs structural building blocks for many tissues and chemical messengers called hormones. They are essential to the proper functioning of the body. So essential are they, in fact, that the body manufactures all the cholesterol building blocks it needs every day. They are integrated into nerve tissue to speed nerve conduction. They are used in the adrenal gland and become chemical, blood-borne messengers to various tissues. They are even the building blocks for the sex hormones, which cause the secondary sexual characteristics (i.e., facial hair in men, breast development in women).

When the body has too much fat in the diet (or because of rare genetic errors of metabolism of fat), it is not used in the normal way, it is changed into cholesterol. The cholesterol is transported through the bloodstream in large amounts, via proteins, to the tissues. Using the heart as an example, the bad cholesterol (LDL) "sticks" abnormally to cells in the artery wall. Over time, it is incorporated into cells (foam cells) which expand. This causes some small blockage in the artery wall (plaque), and the artery tries to dilate to compensate. Initially this compensation is successful, and blood flow continues unabated.

Eventually the artery cannot compensate (even before blood flow is obstructed). This is the time of the most danger because the pressure on these cells can cause the plaque to "burst" (Figure 3). This occurs when the artery is 40% to 60% blocked, but before blood flow is compromised. A big clot forms, suddenly shutting off the artery, causing "myocardial infarction," or death of a portion of the heart tissue.

However, it is also the time when the artery can recover its full diameter and ability to dilate if the excess cholesterol is removed. The damage is not yet permanent! (This is the function of HDL, the "good cholesterol," mentioned later).

A very lowfat diet (10% or fewer calories from fat) also removes excess cholesterol. This is known as the "threshold effect" and is known to occur well under the 30% fat level (recommended by the American Heart Association). Drugs, in high doses, can also remove plaque. There is some question whether they can restore ability to dilate.

When your doctor checks your blood, he gets a report on several parameters.

The **total cholesterol** can be tested on a random sample (i.e., non-fasting). It should be below 200. It consists of LDL cholesterol, HDL cholesterol, and triglycerides. The medical formula, for those of you who are interested, is:

Total Cholesterol = HDL + LDL + (Triglyceride / 5)

Total cholesterol is not a very accurate or useful measure of risk, simply because it is made up of so many components.

LDL cholesterol is the "bad actor". This is the cholesterol made in the liver, in large amounts, and deposited in the arteries of the heart and other vital organs. The lower the level of LDL, the better. An acceptable level is 100.

There are several kinds of LDL. The worst is "oxidized LDL" which is denser and more atherogenic (causes more disease). We call this the "Bad, bad cholesterol." Attempts to keep LDL in the less harmful form by using "anti - oxidants" have been partially successful. Of course, keeping the body from forming any more LDL (through eating right) is a more successful strategy. There is some evidence that, in certain individuals, atherosclerosis can be reversed even without lowering LDL to 100.

Fibrous Plaque   Plaque Rupture

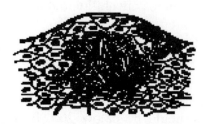 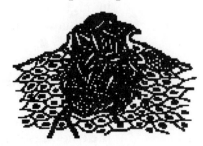

**Figure 3. Over 90% of major myocardial infarcts (> 3 cm)
are associated with plaque ulceration and rupture
(Reference 12)**

<u>**HDL is the "good" cholesterol.**</u> The higher the level, the
better. The HDL transports the bad cholesterol from the
artery wall to the liver where the body can remove it.
Rarely, even when the LDL isn't high, a lack of HDL can
contribute to heart disease (Reference 13). Aerobic exercise,
weight loss, smoking cessation, estrogen replacement after
the menopause and perhaps an alcoholic drink a day can
raise HDL. An acceptable level is 40, but the more, the
better.

> *There is an interesting family in northern Italy.
> Because of a genetic mutation, their HDL
> cholesterol works exceedingly well. Despite their
> diet, (they eat anything and everything they want!)
> they all live well into the ninth decade! If only we
> could all have this gene!*

Some physicians report the ratio of total cholesterol to HDL. The ratio should be 4 or less. This can be useful to calculate risk of heart disease in asymptomatic people if the LDL is not too high and the HDL is not too low. For those with cardiovascular disease, the ratio is meaningless because they already have atherosclerosis. Their cholesterol is already too high for their own good.

Triglycerides are another way the body transports fat through the bloodstream. Although not as directly harmful as LDL, in certain circumstances high triglycerides are a marker for accelerated heart disease. Diabetics can have high levels of triglycerides. At very high levels, pancreatitis (painful inflammation of the pancreas) can develop and can be recurrent.

To accurately measure triglycerides, the blood test must be done after a twelve hour fast. After eating, triglycerides rise rapidly as the intestines transport the fat in the meal to the liver. An acceptable level of triglycerides is 200; desirable is less than 150 mg. Often, high triglycerides and low HDL are found together. Triglyceride problems are helped by a lowfat, low-alcohol, low-simple sugar eating style.

If there is inadequate control of LDL over time, the deposits in the arteries continue to build. The artery can no longer compensate, and blood flow decreases. Although the body tries to form **collateral** blood vessels, frequently they are not adequate, and angina pectoris (chest pressure with exertion) develops. (Collateral blood vessels are new, smaller, parallel blood channels that can grow in number and size in response to stress.) Another factor causing angina is the inability of the artery to dilate.

A heart attack with blood clot may occur in the diseased artery. However, most heart attacks of a serious nature occur when the plaque, and the obstruction to blood flow, is relatively **small**. This used to be reported on angiogram tests as "minimal or insignificant" atherosclerosis. Why does this seemingly contradictory situation happen? The rapid and toxic buildup of the "bad, bad cholesterol" in the artery wall poisons its function. The wall weakens, and as soon as the blood touches these cracks in the wall, a blood clot forms.

Prevention revolves around decreasing LDL (and increasing HDL), by eliminating the fat in the diet, because FAT = CHOLESTEROL. The immediate benefits of a very lowfat diet on angina and heart attack risk are that the arteries dilate more easily and the blood can flow smoothly without slowing or clotting. This happens within two weeks!

One more thought on food and cholesterol. Sooner or later you will have to decide if you want to live to eat, or if you want to eat to live. It is that type of choice with heart disease. If you decide you want to eat to live, you will have to gather the people, places, and things around you that you live for, and count on them as a source of support. Make the choice wisely. MAKE THE CHANGE!

HIGH BLOOD PRESSURE / HYPERTENSION--THE SILENT KILLER

Hypertension, or high blood pressure, occurs when the arteries (outside of the heart arteries) constrict. This raises the pressure needed by the heart to pump blood. The causes of high blood pressure are many. Atherosclerosis can harden the arteries. Poor kidney function can cause hormone messages that raise the pressure. And there are many instances when doctors cannot find the cause.

Side effects of hypertension are deadly (thus, the **silent killer**). It is the most important risk factor for stroke and is high on the list for heart attack, heart failure, and kidney failure. "But, I've always heard that blood pressure should rise with age" you say. However, further research has proven the higher the blood pressure, at any age, the higher the risk of complications (Reference 14).

Therapy begins with weight loss, exercise, and a low salt diet. These have proven of great benefit. Stress and alcohol can cause hypertension to worsen and can be changed to help lower blood pressure. A low salt diet may even help prevent osteoporosis. However, for whatever reason, these instructions are seldom followed even though they have no side effects.

Most therapy consists of drugs, of which there are many. The several classes of drugs consist of: ACE inhibitors, which work in the kidney; Calcium channel blockers, which primarily work on the blood vessels, but also in the heart; diuretics or water pills, which cause the kidneys to get rid of excess water; and beta blockers which slow the heart rate and dilate blood vessels. These all work to some degree. But they may have side effects which limit use. Recently, information on the deleterious side effect of calcium channel blockers has been reported by the news media (Reference 15).

The systolic blood pressure, the top number, is measured when the heart contracts. The diastolic blood pressure, or bottom number, is measured as the heart relaxes. An acceptable blood pressure is 110-120 (systolic) over 60-80 (diastolic). Even lower pressures can be normal as long as there is no associated weakness or dizziness.

DIABETES

Diabetes mellitus is a common disorder of sugar metabolism. The childhood or early onset type is probably genetic or viral in origin and affects younger people. This type is rare and requires very complicated, intensive insulin therapy. This will not be discussed further.

By far the more common type is adult onset diabetes. Although partially genetic, this usually is discovered in older people as they gain weight. Interestingly, with the proper amount of weight loss, 60% to 75% of adult type diabetics can be cured! Although both types share a high blood sugar level, the similarity ends there. The adult type is caused by insulin resistance and high insulin levels. Excess levels of body fat make this possible.

Why all the fuss? Diabetes is a devastating disease, with many serious complications. Remember Harry on page 18? Diabetes is known to accelerate the atherosclerosis process. Also, many diabetics have a co-existing cholesterol (lipid) abnormality, which can be very resistant to therapy. There is a particularly serious combination of diabetes, hypertension, and high lipids which causes complications in the heart at a very high rate (Syndrome X). Diabetics also have a very high rate of vascular disease in the kidneys, legs, and eyes. This can cause gangrene and amputation in the legs, blindness, and kidney failure.

Therapy should be weight reduction. This can cure the disease. However, many do not lose the weight. Then, sugar lowering drugs are used. Unfortunately, although they lower the sugar, they frequently stimulate the appetite. The cycle then repeats itself, i.e., hunger, weight gain, higher sugar, and the need for ever increasing doses of drug. When the **oral hypoglycemic** drugs (pills to lower blood sugar) no longer work, shots of insulin are used. Besides the unpleasantness of once or twice daily injections, the same destructive cycle of hunger, weight gain, and increased dosage can occur. With the epidemic of "American diet" obesity, there are growing numbers of diabetics, all at potential risk of **accelerated atherosclerosis** causing vascular disease in various organs of the body.

A normal blood sugar is from 85 to 100, usually taken in the fasting state. Occasionally a Glucose Tolerance Test is needed to confirm diabetes. This helps make the diagnosis of diabetes if the fasting sugar is normal.

Dan was adamant. "I'm not going to live with this! My father and grandfather died of diabetes. Help me!" With a blood sugar of over 300, sugar in the urine, high cholesterol, and fatigue, Dan needed some help.

Luckily, Dan was serious about not living with his diabetes. He had the common adult onset type. A recent weight gain of thirty pounds, combined with skipping his exercise program because of the job, brought out his diabetes. Dan sat down with his family and decided what was really important. The whole family decided to take daily walks. His wife supported his decision to get on a very lowfat eating plan.

When he returned in a month, Dan felt great! He was no longer fatigued. Even though his sugar was not yet normal, it had dropped by half. And he lost 15 pounds. On his two month visit, at his ideal weight, his blood sugar was normal. As is common, as the sugar came down, so did the cholesterol. "All I really needed was to rethink my priorities. What good is it to make a little more, if I can't watch my kids grow up?"

EXERCISE

Television has the ability to greatly expand our lives. Most of us remember the day that John F. Kennedy was killed because most of us were watching television. Unfortunately, that habit is so ingrained that it has replaced exercise for most Americans.

The great majority of Americans are sedentary. For most, exercise consists of bending over to pick up the morning paper. This contributes to obesity, another American epidemic. Also, it contributes to physical decline and disuse, (mistaken for aging in the past). In other words, **if you don't use it, you lose it**. This goes for heart function, breathing capacity, muscle strength, and mental capacity as well as sexual ability.

There used to be quite a debate about "fitness" versus "health," causing many experts to advocate more extreme methods of exercise than necessary (the marathon craze). However, recent research has proven that even low levels of exercise can reduce the risk of heart disease, stroke, obesity, and joint pain. These levels are the equivalent of walking most every day for 30 minutes. **The most important**

benefits of exercise occur when the otherwise inactive start any exercise, no matter how limited.

There are other benefits of exercise which the sedentary miss. After an exercise session, the appetite is suppressed for several hours. In addition, the metabolism (that favorite excuse of the overweight) is stimulated to a higher level. Often, people will comment on the satisfying mental relaxation that exercise brings. It is certainly a time which can be used for thought, reflection, planning, and rest of the mind. It decreases depression and stress. It makes insulin work more efficiently. Exercise is the most important factor to keep weight off once it is lost.

The benefits of exercise are not related to age. Recent studies in 80-year-olds have shown remarkable improvements in strength, endurance and ability to concentrate. Exercise also helps to prevent falls, the precursor to hip fractures in the elderly.

Sedentary people have more hypertension, obesity, and diabetes. They "age" faster that their active counterparts. They often feel less productive and creative on the job. People who are more active have less fatigue, more energy and sleep better. **<u>Start moving!</u>**

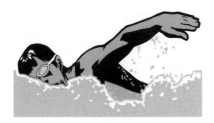

Many people with pre-existing joint problems feel that it hurts too much to exercise, or that it is too tiring. New advances such as water aerobics, water walking, and non-weight bearing machines (i.e, bike) can allow people with these problems to become active and stay active. If you devote at least six weeks to exercise, you will notice the beneficial effects on mood, energy, vigor, weight, and endurance.

Many beginners complain of fatigue. This may often be stress. Exercisers often note a lower stress level, which varies with the duration of their program. Some people with heart disease fear that exercise will hurt them, The opposite is true! Exercise to enhance your longevity.

I'll mention more on starting, and staying with, an exercise program in chapter 9.

SMOKING

Nicotine is the single most addictive substance known to man. The nicotine in tobacco is more addictive than cocaine, alcohol or heroin. No knowledgeable person will say that quitting is easy. But if you have heart disease **you cannot smoke!**

Smoking kills more Americans than alcohol, AIDS, automobiles, and guns combined--every single year. Smoking causes **accelerated atherosclerosis** by a direct effect of the carbon monoxide on the lining cells of the arteries. Smoking also causes direct vasoconstriction (narrowing) of heart arteries, just like cocaine. It causes more sludging and clotting. It causes many types of cancer (see chapter 13, Cancer Prevention). Smoking causes bad breath, emphysema, chronic bronchitis, yellow fingernails, old and wrinkled skin. Smoking kills the sense of smell and the sense of taste and robs you of the enjoyment of food and drink.

It is hard to quit. Prepare several days in advance (see chapter 10 on preparing to quit). Your doctor can help with nicotine patches. You can chew gum, change your routine, cut down on caffeine (to lessen your nervousness and anxiety), and send your clothes to the dry cleaners. The worst of the withdrawal will be over in two weeks, but experienced abstainers know that the urge will last a lifetime. (It's like coveting thy neighbor's wife--it's what you do with the urge that counts). Replace the habit with a new hobby, one that you can do 20-30-40 times a day, instead of lighting up. **<u>DO NOT SMOKE!</u>**

Stress may increase during withdrawal, but then it will plummet to new lows as you free yourself from the slavery of nicotine!

Yes, you may experience a transient weight gain. This lasts from 60-90 days, and can be lessened by exercise. Your health will improve, even if you gain a few pounds.

Learn more on kicking the habit in chapter 10.

AGE

Age is an interesting risk factor. The more years you lead an excessive lifestyle with an overabundance of fat, food, and smoke, and a paucity of exercise, the more atherosclerosis you will have. Studies from the examination of childhood car accident victims have proven that fatty streaks in the aorta (the major blood vessel from the heart) begin by the age of ten. Studies of wartime casualties have proven that atherosclerosis is well established by the age of twenty. Studies of athletes have proven that the major cause of sudden death over the age of 35 is coronary artery disease! It is no wonder that, as we age, an increasing number of complications develop in the cardiovascular system, simply due to the passage of time and the work of risk factors.

Women past the menopause have accelerated atherosclerosis. The special problems of women will be addressed in chapter 7.

FAMILY HISTORY

The medical history of heart disease in immediate family members can act as a marker for various problems, such as cholesterol disorders, possibly of a genetic nature. When the family has premature heart disease (under age 55), this is an additional risk factor. This deserves intense consideration because it raises your risk of having the same type of problem. You should help your doctor take a thorough, detailed medical family history.

STRESS

I love stories with a happy ending! I also see many people, like Clair, who start out miserable. We started out talking about smoking. She wanted to quit. It was soon evident that smoking was not the main problem.

"I'm cold. I can't relate to my husband or our friends. I just don't enjoy life like I used to!" Then the tears came. "I can't control anything in my life, my emotions, eating, sleeping, anything. I used to love life. Now I don't feel anything at all." As it turned out, these feelings had surfaced, once before, just after high school graduation. But with a new job, new boyfriend, and a different outlook, the situation quickly resolved.

There were major problems among Clair's family. She and her husband hadn't had sex in months. He was working longer, and she didn't care. Their oldest was acting up in school, and his grades were falling. His mouth was acting up at home, too. Clair just wanted to rest.

There were many instances of depression in Clair's relatives. Her father had been treated. He advised her to get some help. We discussed the situation for a long time. Because she was already feeling helpless, it took Clair a while to decide what to do. Finally, we agreed to arrange counseling and try an anti-depressant.

This was a big step for Clair. But she was determined to break out of her "funk." And when she returned several weeks later, she did feel better. "Finally, I can sleep. I'm not great, but my mind behaves me now. When I feel sad, I cry, but I can feel happy, too. I can laugh again."It took three months, but she changed. Life had meaning. She sought new challenges in school. The love between Clair and her husband deepened. Quitting the nicotine habit went well. Her new job made her feel useful to herself and others. She told me how she appreciated the way she now functioned. "I never, ever want to feel depressed again!"

Our present day society is a killer! The pace of life has increased 10 fold in only the last generation. All the innovations, inventions and labor saving devices have seemingly done the opposite--created less leisure time and more stress. Instead of peace and quiet, our faxes, cellular telephones and pagers find us everywhere. Instead of limits to our work day, our work expands to fill 24 hours.

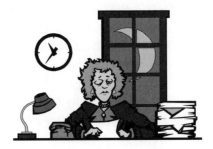

When the human race was in its infancy, we needed to be fleet of foot, strong and determined. The hunter-gatherer life required quick reflexes and speed to run away from enemies or to catch prey. Over the centuries, humans developed the **fight or flight response**. Through a series of hormones (adrenaline and cortisone) transmitted through the bloodstream, our bodies received a quick burst of energy, our blood was shunted to only the most vital organs, and our senses were awakened. In the event of injury, these messages helped us stop bleeding and recuperate. In the event of a fight, the eyesight narrowed to focus on the aggressor, the strength increased, and the reflexes quickened. These responses helped the race to flourish.

Let's fast forward to the twentieth century. Not many of us fight saber toothed tigers anymore. The closest many come to a race may be to catch the morning bus. A confrontation may begin in the boardroom or the bedroom. However, physiology responds as it did in hunter-gatherer times: the elevated blood pressure, constricted arteries and surge of adrenaline which now is not relieved by a fight or flight. The response is left for the body to dissipate while going about sedentary life--answering the phone, driving the car and using the computer. Eventually this bodily over-response catches up, causing hypertension, coronary artery spasm, and maladaptive behaviors. We all know those who over-eat, over-drink, and party excessively, take drugs and smoke. These behaviors may temporarily mask the discomfort of stress but are certainly not the cure.

In modern America more people feel isolated and alone, lonely. We can fool ourselves that staring at the TV or taking a "Love Boat" cruise is social intercourse. However real dialog on feelings and human emotions is lacking in many lives. Some people have simply never learned to effectively communicate and are left with platitudes (how about those Rockies!). Others, because of real or imagined slights, deliberately cut themselves off to avoid more pain. Still others lock themselves into a rigid pattern learned of necessity during a crisis. Many Americans are "disconnected" from the social structure of home, family, work and neighborhood.

Modern Americans live in fear: fear of violence, fear of intimacy, and fear of themselves. The pioneer spirit of adventure, that each day gave a new opportunity, is replaced by the drudgery of routine, joyless chores, tasks to be completed before retiring from life to the world of TV.

Doctors and psychiatrists call these states depression, anxiety, and despair. Also loneliness, drug abuse, and alcoholism. New drugs are often prescribed. However, with sensitivity, communication, and understanding, control of the body, mind and emotions can be regained. This leads to true integration into society and enhanced happiness and well-being. Help close the door on maladaptive behaviors, and open the door to greater health of the body and the mind! When happiness and inner peace lead to empowerment and motivation, great changes are possible.

Others have risen above their foibles, and so can you. Witness the great works in art and literature of people, ordinary people, rising above despair. Use your peers, in a supportive group environment, to do the same.

Please ask your doctor specific questions you may have about your risk factors. They are very important in the quest to prevent heart disease. Knowledge is power, and this knowledge will help you regain power and control over your life.

The old saying, "an ounce of prevention is worth a pound of cure" is true, especially when it comes to your health. Those of you scared because of symptoms, your family history, or a long list of risk factors can benefit from this program. You will also realize a decreased risk of cancer of various causes. Some modifications are possible in those not yet sick, and I will point them out.

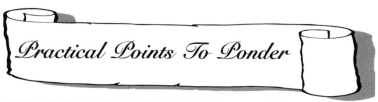

Practical Points To Ponder

HEART DISEASE RISK FACTORS

Hardening of the arteries is an epidemic!

Risk factors cause it. Which of the causes of heart disease do you have the power to change?

- ♥ High cholesterol
- ♥ High blood pressure
- ♥ Diabetes, especially the overweight type
- ♥ Lack of exercise
- ♥ Smoking
- ♥ Age or years with an unhealthy lifestyle
- ♥ Family history or genetics (change your jeans!!)
- ♥ Stress!!!!!!!!

This program is designed for those with proven heart disease. Consider how serious another heart attack would be. If nothing changes in YOUR lifestyle, nothing will change in your disease, or in your health.

The program can easily be adapted by those at risk of disease, or by those wishing to support their loved ones who are already battling for their lives.

HOW MUCH TO CHANGE?

You may take the attitude that a little, gradual change at a time is easier than an all out, all at once revolution. Experience teaches that most people, after a little change, will quickly go back to the original behavior. This could be disastrous! Our advice, during this program, is to **make all the changes at once**, and participate in an ongoing group support system. You've thought about it. You've prepared for it. Now, just do it! In this way, the change in taste of food, the slimmer waist from exercise, and the mental doubts are all combined with the improved physical well-being gained in the first two weeks. Eventually you will have to go all the way; show a sense of commitment and start from the very beginning! (More on change in chapter 8, page 178)

<u>Food for thought:</u>

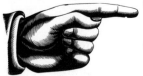

- ♥ You can regain control of your life, health, and happiness.

- ♥ Be a willing, active participant in the change.

- ♥ Think about making all the changes at once. It's easier and more effective than the usual slow torture method.

<u>MAKE THE CHANGE!</u>

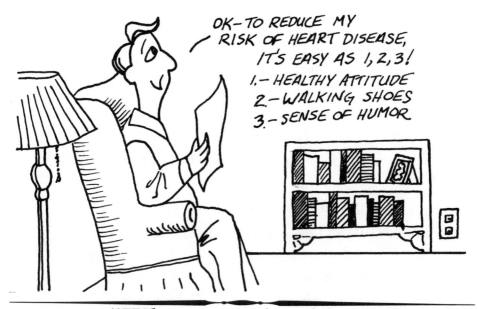

CHAPTER 3

THE PRACTICAL WAY TO REVERSE BLOCKED ARTERIES!

> *"What you should put first in all the practice of your art is how to make the patient well; and if he can be made well in many ways, one should choose the least troublesome."*

Hippocrates

This plan consists of several cornerstones:

♥ Tasty, easily prepared lowfat diet;

♥ Daily exercise;

- ♥ Smoking cessation;
- ♥ Stress reduction;
- ♥ Self-awareness and group support.

They are all equally important, and help you in different ways. The following is a brief summary of the various components of the plan. We will, in other chapters, go into further detail.

MAKE THE CHANGE EATING PLAN

QUESTIONS ABOUT THE EATING PLAN

1. *Won't I tire easily if I don't eat fat?*

   The best source of energy is from carbohydrates, not fat. Excess fat in food turns to the fat you wear (around the waist). Eat carbohydrates to regain energy.

2. *I've heard you can't get complete protein unless you eat meat.*

   There are certain amino acids, the building blocks of proteins, that may not be present at each meal. It was previously thought that you had to combine complimentary proteins at the same meal to have complete protein. (Beans and rice, for example.) However, as long as you eat a variety of foods throughout the day, you will have the correct amount and type of the necessary amino acids.

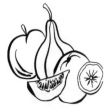

3. **My doctor told me vegetarians don't get enough vitamin B_{12}.**

After about three years, our stores of B_{12} can run down on a vegetarian eating plan. If you don't have a reliable source of B_{12} from fortified foods or skim dairy products, take a B_{12} pill once a month.

4. *Can't a lowfat diet be unhealthy?*

A diet can be unhealthy at any fat level--it depends on your food choices! Most would agree that it's a **high fat** diet that brings on many health problems. By following the Make the Change Meal Plan on page 80 you can be assured a high quality plan for overall good health.

5. *How will I keep from getting hungry if I don't have a cheeseburger for lunch?*

You may indeed have to eat more often on a lowfat meal plan. Low fat foods pass quickly from the stomach. An interesting side effect is the absence of heartburn with a lowfat meal.

6. *Isn't this just for kooks?*

Examination of eating styles of people who eat a lot of meat show high levels of heart disease, cancer, and contaminants such as antibiotics, hormones, and bacteria. True, media advertising pushes the average American to eat beef, chicken and dairy. Media moguls may not be thinking of your health, however. They spend $40 billion a year to advertise their products to you and your kids.

7. *How will I get enough protein on a meatless plan?*

It is surprisingly easy to meet the RDA for protein, even on a meatless meal plan. Many meat eaters eat about twice as much protein as they really need--which causes it's own problems. The bottom line is--if you're eating enough calories, you're probably eating enough protein.

The typical American eats far too much fat for good health (because FAT = CHOLESTEROL). Protein in overabundance can actually cause physical problems. Carbohydrates, the energy food, have been given short shrift. Typical percentages of these foods, in terms of calories: fat 40 - 50%, protein 30 - 40%, and carbohydrates 10 - 30%. Typical "diets" make you hungry, and sometimes put the body into starvation mode, making it hard to burn calories efficiently.

On your new eating plan, fat = 10% or less, protein = 20%, and carbohydrates = 70% or more of calories. Why? It is medically proven that a 5 - 10% fat diet can and does reverse atherosclerosis. The "threshold for reversal" is reached. It is also proven that a 30% American Heart Association diet does **not improve or reverse** atherosclerosis (Reference 16). To test fat levels between 10% and 30% few studies have been done (but people have unique thresholds for reversal). One thing you should not feel is hungry. When fat is eliminated, it opens up the possibility of more **volume** of healthy food. Your stomach and taste buds will not lack stimulation.

THE BUILDING BLOCKS OF FOOD

For recipes, see chapter 14.

FAT

Fat contains 9 calories per gram, which is very calorie intense. Also, dietary fat is efficiently stored in the body, as "cellulite" or "love handles." There are different kinds of fat; however, all have undesirable effects, and all are unhealthy in excess. "You are what you eat" pertains to fat and your love handles!

Monounsaturated fat (found in olive oil or canola oil) has been called "good fat" although it is 14% saturated fat. (It is important to distinguish chemical compounds such as monounsaturated fats from foods such as olive oil. All natural foods which contain fat have some saturated fat.) There is no one "perfect food." See table 1 for breakdown on different oils.

Fat	%Sat	%Poly	%Mono
Canola Oil	6	32	62
Safflower Oil	10	77	13
Sunflower Oil	11	69	20
Corn Oil	13	62	25
Olive Oil	14	9	77
Soybean Oil	15	61	24
Peanut Oil	18	33	49
Chicken Fat	31	22	47
Lard	41	12	47
Beef Fat	52	4	4
Palm Kernel Oil	81	2	11
Coconut Oil	92	2	6

Table 1. Comparison of fats.
(Source: US Department of Agriculture)

Polyunsaturated fat (safflower and corn oil) comes from vegetable sources. Again, the actual foods such as safflower and corn oil have some saturated fat.

Saturated fat is the undisputed worst for health. It is directly linked to production of LDL, the "bad cholesterol." Saturated fat comes mostly from animal sources, but is found in high amounts in coconut and palm oils and chocolate.

Synthetic fat is chemically treated, turning it into "trans" fatty acids which have a long shelf life, but correspondingly shorten **your** life. These are frequently listed on labels as "partially hydrogenated vegetable oils," often found in margarine and shortening.

Recent research in the Journal of the National Cancer Institute proves that men on a high fat diet suffer an increased risk of **prostate cancer** (Reference 17). Women suffer higher rates of **breast cancer** (Reference 18). Both sexes have more **colon cancer** with the high fat American style diet.

How many grams of fat do we need each day? Probably only 5 grams (2% of calories) daily to meet our nutritional requirements. How many calories in a pound of fat? We need to burn about 3500 calories to loose a pound of pure fat. This equates to 10 - 14 days of walking 30 minutes at a good pace. How many grams of fat do typical Americans eat, each day? About 100 grams--20 times more than the minimum!

Most of the fat in American food comes from four main sources: animal muscle (meat, chicken, and fish); dairy products (milk, cheese, ice cream); baked goods (pies, cakes, cookies); and condiments (gravy, salad dressing, sour cream). These are discouraged on your new meal plan. The other sources of fat are mostly from vegetable sources, such as nuts, avocados, soybeans, and tofu. What are not healthy are synthetic fats, usually found in off-the-shelf baked goods.

The minimal amount of fat ingested on the new meal plan will insure the fastest reversal of atherosclerosis possible. Improvement can start in two weeks! For those with established heart disease, this is also the safest course to follow. For those with pre-existing heart disease, no amount of saturated fat is safe to eat.

> *I'd like to illustrate what a very lowfat intake can do. A general surgeon, Dr. Stanley Dudrick, put patients, deathly ill with angina and coronary blockages, on a "water" diet. Then, through an IV, he "fed" them a solution of amino acids (which are the building blocks of protein) and sugar for 90 days. The angina disappeared, blood flow increased, the patients got out of their wheelchairs and began to lead a normal life (Reference 19).*

> *When they started to eat solid foods again the blockage rapidly returned because they hadn't learned to limit the fat in their diet. I know, this approach sounds drastic, but it is an example of proven, rapid results by getting rid of fat.*

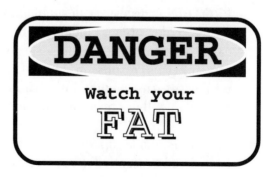

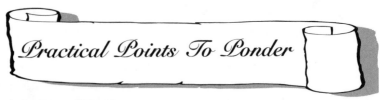

Practical Points To Ponder

FOOD TIPS

- ♥ There is no one "perfect food"

- ♥ Moderation is relative, says Lynn Fischer, author of The Low Cholesterol Gourmet. "A guy has half a baked potato with sour cream. He eats half of his asparagus with hollandaise. He eats half of his raspberry pie with ice cream. And he eats half of his steak. He's hungry and he's had 1,000 grams of saturated fat and 1,000 milligrams of cholesterol." (Reference 20).

- ♥ One day a month, give yourself permission to eat anything and everything you desire. This reduces the daily urge to "cheat."

PROTEIN

PROTEIN is necessary in small amounts for the structure of all the major organs, including muscle. Many "pop" diets can produce a rapid weight loss, caused by loss of water and protein. This results in loss of muscle and subsequent weakness. Any weight loss originating from your lowfat meal plan will not result in these undesirable consequences.

Protein is made up of amino acids, nine of which are considered "essential" (they need to be consumed in food). The other amino acids can be made in the body, from the basic building blocks, and used as needed to build tissue. There used to be a controversy surrounding "complete" protein, some contending that animal products were necessary to form complete protein. Rest assured, this has been debunked. As a matter of fact, rice and beans together produce all the essential amino acids, and just eating a variety of food throughout the day supplies all the "complete" proteins the body needs.

Another source of controversy is the overabundance of protein in the typical American diet. Researchers have implicated loss of protein by-products through the urine, linked with loss of calcium, as one cause of osteoporosis (the epidemic disease of older women which leaches the strength from bones, causing the "dowager hump" and hip fractures). The type of protein (animal vs. soy) also seems to affect calcium balance. (Reference 21)

The average man needs only about 50 grams of protein a day; women about 44 grams a day. (RDA's are higher than average needs. Recent research shows that some older people may need more protein than the RDA (Reference 22).) One cup of navy beans has 15 grams of protein, 1 cup noodles 7 grams, and 1 cup skim milk has 9 grams with virtually no fat. Compare this to 3 1/2 ounces. of lean ground beef which has 24 grams of protein, plus 18 grams of fat. The added bonus of protein--only 4 calories per gram.

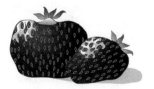
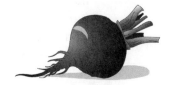

SOURCES OF PROTEIN IN FOODS

Food item	Grams of Protein
Tofu, 1/2 cup raw firm	20
Lentils, 1 cup cooked	18
Pinto beans, 1 cup	14
Soybeans, 1/2 cup	14
Quinoa, 1/2 cup cooked	11
Yogurt, vanilla nonfat 1 cup	10
Split pea soup, 1 cup	9
Skim milk, 1 cup	8
Soy milk, 1 cup	7
Most grains and vegetables, 1 serving	2-3

Table 2. Protein in Foods

CARBOHYDRATES

CARBOHYDRATES are the energy food. Carbos are very efficiently converted to energy in muscle, causing increased muscular endurance. They contain only 4 calories per gram, allowing you to partake often.

Carbos come in many forms. Simple carbos (one molecule) are sugar. They are also called "empty calories" because they don't contain other nutrients, such as vitamins and minerals. (On the other hand, they don't have any fat either.) Many foods taste sweet because of added sugar, a good example being breakfast cereal. Those of you who count calories, beware of simple sugar for two reasons: the calorie count goes up, and our dental colleagues tell us they cause cavities. In some sensitive individuals, and especially in diabetics, too many simple sugars can cause a rise in triglycerides.

Complex carbos are known as starches. Complex carbos are absorbed slowly and are better for the metabolism. They tend to even out the blood sugar, protecting us from wide swings (hypoglycemia). Those with triglyceride problems do better with complex rather than simple carbos. When muscles are fatigued, complex carbos in the form of "sports drinks" (weak solution of complex carbos) are the most efficient replenishment. Additionally, complex carbos affect the metabolism, causing food to be burned off as energy efficiently, and not stored as fat. (Carbos have a high **specific dynamic action**. This means that carbos are used quickly and the process costs the body energy to do this).

Fiber is a long chain of sugars, so long the body doesn't have enzymes to break it up. They are passed, unchanged, in the feces. They do attract water into the colon, speeding up the movement of food products through the colon and relieving constipation. This cures many rectal problems, such as hemorrhoids and rectal itch.

The greatest benefit of fiber, however, is the prevention of colon cancer. In countries where the colon cancer rate is low, the diet contains over 30 grams of fiber a day. Americans, with an average fiber intake of about 5-10 grams a day, have a much higher rate of colon cancer. Your new meal plan should have 30 grams of fiber. For the first weeks, this may take some adjustment: some experience gas or bloating initially on a high fiber diet. This will not harm you, but colon cancer can harm and even kill you. Read more on cancer prevention in chapter 13.

Fiber prevents diverticulosis, inhibits polyp formation, and relieves constipation. It also makes bowel movements easy to pass, eliminating straining. See list of high fiber food page 244.

Please see the chapter 4 list of **healthy foods**, which improve diabetes, lower blood pressure, and help you attain your optimal weight. These foods have a positive health benefit. Fatty foods, as you now know, have a negative health benefit.

VITAMINS are important chemical compounds which help the metabolic activity of the body. They are required, in certain amounts, for health. The fat soluble vitamins, those are stored by the body, are A, D, E, and K. They are available in a healthy meal plan such as you are starting.

ANTIOXIDANTS

ProVitamin A (beta-carotene) is an **antioxidant**. When certain compounds (for example, LDL, the bad cholesterol) are damaged by chemical reactions in the body, an antioxidant can delay or abort this damage (Reference 23). Beta-carotene (25,000 IU daily) has been proven to have beneficial effects on health, both cancer AND heart attack prevention.

Foods with large amounts of beta-carotene include carrots, sweet potatoes, spinach, broccoli, cantaloupes, apricots, and asparagus.

Vitamin E is also an antioxidant. In doses up to 400 IU daily, it has been proven to have a beneficial effect on heart disease, probably by delaying or aborting the oxidation of

LDL. In the dose needed to prevent heart disease, this may be the only vitamin you should supplement.

Vitamin C is another antioxidant, readily available in fruits. It has been proven to have an anti-cancer effect. A dose of 1,000 to 2,000 mg. a day is sufficient.

Nutrient	Dose	Effect
Vitamin E	400 IU	Reduce Heart Disease
Beta Carotene	25 mg. or 25,000 IU	Reduce Heart Disease and Cancer
Vitamin C	1,000 mg.	Helps Vitamin E work

Table 3. Antioxidants

Present studies say these amounts work; doses may vary depending on individual requirements.

There is a comprehensive discussion of vitamins and minerals in chapter 11.

MINERALS AND OTHER NUTRIENTS

MINERALS are essential to the proper functioning of the body. They are non-organic substances that aid the chemical reactions of the body in different ways.

Calcium is essential, not only to the bones and teeth, but also for the proper regulation of blood flow in the arteries. It is found in green, leafy vegetables, legumes, nuts, whole grains and dairy products. There is quite a controversy surrounding the calcium in dairy foods. Because of the large amounts of protein in our diets (a large portion coming from milk and animal protein), the kidneys may excrete more calcium than is taken in (Reference 24 and and reference 25). Therefore, a lower protein diet, like recommended in Make The Change, will help you achieve optimum calcium balance. Calcium pills are available, but absorption of calcium is higher in food than pills, so it is best to get your calcium from nonfat sources like high calcium vegetables or nonfat dairy products. See page 154 for Calcium and osteoporosis and page 156 food sources of calcium.

Sodium and chloride combine to make **salt**, as in table salt. They are essential to the proper functioning of the nerves, in fluid balance, and in acid-base balance. The typical American diet has 50 to 100 times the salt needed. Too much salt can lead to hypertension, edema, or swelling, as well as osteoporosis.

Iron is used in the hemoglobin molecule in the red blood cell. This carries oxygen around the body. **Too much iron, especially in men, has been implicated in heart disease**. Women seem to suffer less than men from heart disease caused by iron overload.

There are many other nutrients, all available on your new meal plan, which are not only essential, but serve to protect against various cancers. The typical American diet may sometimes be deficient in these nutrients because of lack of variety, a low fruit and vegetable intake, and over-processing. These substances, called **phytochemicals**, can protect against cancer. They are found in cabbage, broccoli, brussels sprouts, cauliflower, greens, horseradish, garlic, and soybeans and more. Some phytochemicals, which are undiscovered, may be present in food, but absent from pills. It seems prudent to eat right, even if you consider using a supplement, see chapter 11 for more information.

A word about water. Water flushes the body of chemicals, helping to insure good kidney function. In combination with fiber, it helps form soft, easy-to-pass bowel movements. It can even help edema (swelling) by allowing the kidney to excrete excess sodium. Water can act as a natural appetite suppressant (if you desire), when taken cold and just prior to meals. Water can also act as a substitute for more harmful drinks, such as those containing too much caffeine (or other stimulants) or too much alcohol (or other depressants).

I'll answer your questions about supplements in detail in chapter 11.

CONDIMENTS

Lest you think your food will not stimulate your taste buds, be sure to have lots of condiments on hand. Some suggestions:

- ♥ No-salt seasonings, barbecue sauce (low sodium, oil free), fruit jams (pure fruit, no sugar), maple syrup, Dijon mustard, fat-free salad dressing, salsa (low sodium, oil free), Tabasco sauce, ketchup, and Worcestershire sauce.

- ♥ Most herbs and spices can be added to taste. Also, don't forget lemon juice, honey, vinegar, and various fresh and dried fruits.

- ♥ Many spices lose their flavor after a year. Be sure to keep your spices and other flavorings up to date, to appreciate the true flavor of your cuisine!

I'll help you set up your kitchen in chapter 5.

OFF THE SHELF FOODS

For those not used to cooking at home, many new low and no fat choices are now available. See chapter 4, chapter 5, and chapter 6 for all the details.

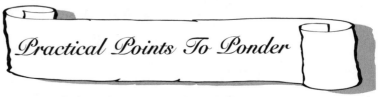

Practical Points To Ponder

MANAGE YOUR STRESS

- ♥ If you will learn to manage stress better, you will be able to take control of your life.
- ♥ Exercise is the best short term stress reducer.
- ♥ Spend five minutes writing down the things that are most important in your life. Compare that with the things you spend most of your time doing. Cut back if you are doing things that aren't important.
- ♥ Join a group, any group!
- ♥ Use the power of love, whether in a religious, platonic, or romantic sense, to get you through the hard times.

STRESS MANAGEMENT

Stress! We all live with it on a daily basis. Some people have a very visible reaction to stress such as wringing hands and pacing. They proclaim loudly, "I'm stressed out!" Others, however, seem to internalize stress. Outwardly calm, they seethe on the inside. Chest pain, headaches, diarrhea and belly pain cause no change in their demeanor. Why is this?

Stress consists of so many different factors. To some, it is isolation, depression, and physical disabilities. A typical high stress group consists of elderly white males. Research shows they have three times more likelihood of committing suicide than non-white males and six times more incidence of committing suicide than females.

In many societies, the elders are revered, sought after for their wisdom. Not so in America. Here, nursing homes and retirement communities are a growth industry. Social isolation is an American epidemic with many causes: fear of crime, television addiction, poor communication skills, and unwillingness to change.

There are several habits we can utilize to end social isolation. The classic method is to not be alone: get a pet, join a club, volunteer time in the hospital nursery or pediatric ward. In addition, **communication skills can be improved**. There are several methods:

- ♥ The easiest to master is the art of listening, then briefly repeating in your own words what was said. Especially in emotionally charged situations, such as with family, this method can be helpful. It tends to slow down and focus verbal communication, and enhances "body language" or non-verbal communication.

- ♥ Another communication skill to master is that of speaking about feelings rather than thoughts. We spend a lifetime learning to "edit" before we speak, making assumptions (or guesses) which may be incorrect. These usually are spoken as "thoughts." "I think you are angry" and "I think you need to rest" are examples of speaking thoughts. In times of stress, try speaking feelings, such as "I am angry, happy, embarrassed, lonely, worried, insecure, or sad." Then ask your loved one to respond similarly. (No fair trying "I feel you need a psychiatrist"!). This method can help get to the root of the situation or problem, thus opening up discussion based on the real issue. At the very least, it will clean up the line of communication, so that both parties are "on the same wavelength." It takes openness and practice to speak feelings, and this, too, indicates willingness to have a dialog rather than the usual shouting match.

For some other ideas on stress, Refer to "Thirty-five Ways to Leave your Stress" in chapter 8.

ANXIETY is commonly reported to cause distress and lack of satisfaction. In contemporary society there is much to make us anxious. Anxiety can escalate to the point of discomfort, causing withdrawal from many social situations, which is not good for mental health. It can also be frightening, as the symptoms of an anxiety or panic attack can mimic heart attack, with chest pressure, shortness of breath, rapid heart beat, and sweating.

Besides medication, there are several helpful techniques which alleviate anxiety. **The quieting response** (see chapter 8) is effective to physically use reflexes to relax both the body and the mind. **The body stress scanning** technique (also chapter 8) is also effective. We urge you to learn and practice both these techniques often.

There is a group of behaviors, termed "learned behavior" (or **Type A behavior**), that seem to trap people on the treadmill of work. Often initiated at an early age (some experts say inborn), the typical pattern is a relentless, unyielding work ethic. Pretty good for business, you say. However, after the first couple of years of accomplishment, praise, promotion, and reward, these people don't seem to be able to "slow down and smell the roses." Often there is tension between spouses, but the Type A may not understand why (even after the umpteenth missed dinner). Life to them seems to be competition, and slowing down or vacationing means falling behind. They thrive on pressure, deadlines, and challenges. Some, when the inevitable heart attack comes, don't want to be hospitalized, or after the first day begin to doubt they need care (i.e., I must have had bad heartburn!). Occasionally, the Type A will insist on doing push-ups at the bedside, while hooked up to the monitor, to prove everything is OK!

There is more to life than work, even for the long-term Type A personality. Often the best therapy is a close examination of goals. However, before this can be accomplished, the merry-go-round must stop.

Strange as it may seem, there are few of us who have complete control of our own minds. With practice, the worries, schedules and demands that keep the mind working in overtime can be pushed out. Control of the mind during meditation allows for relaxation of the body, also. Relaxation and control. Together, they bring peace of mind (or inner peace). Many find it easier to discern the true goals in their lives after meditation. Hopefully, you will be able to reflect on your goals and desires in a constructive way.

ANGER is often found in people with heart or other serious disease. It is as if, instead of screaming, these people keep anger inside, till they (and their arteries) burst. Anger can and does come out eventually, but often is aimed inappropriately at the ones closest to us. Anger is a strong emotion. Anger can also mask depression. Many are afraid of it because it is so strong. Talking about anger, directing it appropriately, and understanding where it came from sometimes help it be released, from inside. This can be a very gratifying experience. More about anger and how to deal with it is available in chapter 8.

FATIGUE is a symptom of many things: burn-out, insomnia, inability to cope, and depression. Sometimes it simply comes from prolonged physical inactivity.

DEPRESSION is very detrimental to high level functioning, in business and at home. This unfortunate disease can be a block to reaching your goals: happiness, health, vigor, love. Depression drags down the mind and body. It actually inhibits the normal functioning of body tissues. Other symptoms of depression are change in appetite, insomnia, inability to feel pleasure, helplessness and hopelessness. Depression is a common ailment, affecting up to 20% of Americans. If this sounds like you, let your personal physician know. There are many treatments which can help you remove this blockage, and help you heal the blockage in your heart. Read about them in chapter 8. The treatment is available, and it works. There is no reason to continue to feel this way!

It is a fact of our modern American society that many women and men have been **victimized** sexually, physically, and emotionally. This can leave deep scars and memories, some of which may not even be conscious. This can adversely affect us in our later years as the "scars" open up. Many of these attributes are found in victims; in fact, heart disease may bring them out into the open. Maladaptive behavior, learned to cope with prior abuse, is often used to endure. By recognizing that the abuse was actual, and real, and then (thankfully) leaving it in the past, present day happiness and peace can be a realistic goal.

The stress reduction component of our program would not be complete without group support. We spend several hours a week in our group at the Preventive Health Institute. It can be a valuable learning and healing tool. Group support can be as straightforward as an invitation to a fat-free meal! Often, groups evolve into "networks" for exercise and social life. Some even take the step of giving counsel and love to members in distress. Don't forget that word, love. It can be a lifesaver. Freud said, "the purpose of life is to love and to work." Many great philosophers and religious leaders have recognized the power of love to overcome obstacles. Don't downplay love's ability to get you through.

You are urged to join group sessions in your community. None available, you say? Write the Preventive Health Institute for information on how to start a group. Others have found this the single most helpful intervention they can make in their lifestyle.

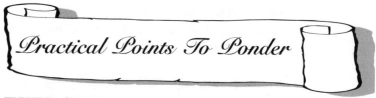

Practical Points To Ponder

EXERCISE!

♥ "No pain, no gain" is a myth. If you hurt, see your doctor. Something may be wrong.

- ♥ The most danger from an exercise program is at the very beginning. Be careful! Start out low and slow and gradually build up.

- ♥ Aerobic exercise should be a priority to prevent and reverse heart disease. Strength training is fine if you have more time.

- ♥ Most people settle on walking for 30 minutes most every day. Variety is the spice of life, so have a backup if you feel stale or the weather turns ugly. Try swimming, rowing, or biking for variety!

- ♥ At times during this program, the expense and side - effects of your medicines may begin to outweigh the benefits. This is especially true for blood pressure, sugar, and cholesterol medicines. The good effects of exercise, low-fat food, and stress reduction may make them less necessary. Please keep in touch with your personal physician, and discuss any changes in your medicine before you change them on your own.

EXERCISE--MOVE YOUR BODY

Most of "aging" is really disuse. As the saying goes, "if you don't use it, you lose it." This is true, but you can gain some of it back. This takes exercise, however, about 30 minutes most every day.

Learn how to exercise the easy way in chapter 9.

Exercise can help your heart in several ways. The muscles of the extremities, with daily use, develop greater capacity to pull oxygen from the blood. The mitochondria (power plants) of the muscle hypertrophy, and the muscle becomes more efficient (At this stage of life, don't expect to see too much enlargement of your muscles). This causes beneficial effects in energy and vigor, even without any changes in the heart.

In addition, exercise will affect the heart and lungs. Weight loss will make it easier to move. Just as for other muscles, the heart and diaphragm muscles will respond by becoming more efficient (mitochondria multiply). The heart benefits directly by having more oxygen supply. Although you should notice beneficial effects within two weeks, it is extremely important to **start low and go slow**. Most people overdo the first day. When they wake up the next day, soreness causes them to call off the whole program. Remember, you are in this for the long haul. This is called **pleasurable** risk reduction.

STRETCHING can help prevent soreness. It is also important as a warm-up. This slowly stimulates the heart, allowing compensation to occur. (For those of you with angina pectoris, you know the initial morning walk can bring it on. Then, after a rest and compensation occur, exercise can continue for much longer without symptoms.) The best resource is "Stretching" by Bob Anderson. Try several stretches, very slowly

When your muscles are warmed up, it is time to start the aerobic part of exercise. (See chapter 9, for the exact "exercise prescription.") Eventually try to work up to 30 minutes most every day, but initially, remember to **start low and go slow**. Follow the parameters of the exercise prescription. Many people settle on walking as the optimal exercise because of convenience, but feel free to experiment with other equipment or sports. Water sports are a good alternative, especially if arthritis, weight, or weather are factors.

The last part of the exercise program is the cool-down. As the body exercises, blood vessels dilate and "energizing" (fight or flight) hormones are released. The cool down allows these changes to reverse slowly. Some exercisers get dizzy if they skip the cool down. The main reason for the cool-down, though, is to avoid changes in the rhythm of the heart (arrhythmias) from the high levels of hormones.

Many people are afraid that exercise, especially after a heart attack, will hurt them. While it is prudent to start low and slow, your heart, body, and mind desperately need exercise. Far from causing harm, exercise strengthens the heart and helps longevity. Use it or lose it!

If you have adverse effects from exercise, modifications can be made immediately. "Warnings" (chapter 9) can be used as a guide. Most people will notice 1-2 weeks of a not unpleasant relaxation when they start an exercise program. This soon changes into a phase of increased energy and vigor, which will stay with you as long as you continue the program. The rise in **endorphins** causes these positive mental and physical benefits.

Most complaints about exercise are about time. It is suggested to pick a time of day and stick to it. Form a habit. Practice, practice, practice. Soon it will be a routine part of your day, like eating and sleeping.

Look for further suggestions in chapter 9, the practical way to start an exercise program.

CHAPTER 4

EATING RIGHT, THE PRACTICAL GUIDE

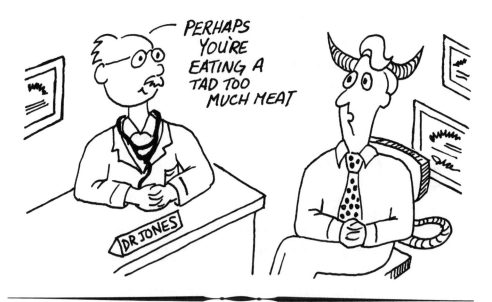

PERHAPS YOU'RE EATING A TAD TOO MUCH MEAT

DR JONES

"You are what you eat."

WHAT YOU WILL FIND IN THIS CHAPTER

- ♥ Keeping the vitamins in your food (page 88)
- ♥ Recipe Substitutions (page 89)
- ♥ In Place of Meat: where is the beef? (page 93)
- ♥ Beans about Beans (page 95)
- ♥ Short cuts to Vegetarian Eating (page 97)
- ♥ Recipe Make-overs (page 99)
- ♥ Controlling the Hunger Monster (page 103)

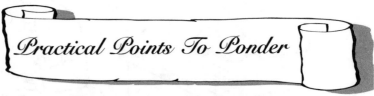

Practical Points To Ponder

TEN STEPS TO HEALTHY EATING

1. Have a clear idea of your overall goal. Give up one cheeseburger a week? Expect very slight improvement. **Big change, big improvement!**

2. Have a clear idea which foods contain fat. Read the section on **food labels**, see chapter 5. The Department of Agriculture does not require meat, chicken, or milk products to have labels, yet they are all very high in fat!

3. Test yourself on your **knowledge** of nutrition. (Take the Nutrition Survey next page).

   Aim for a total of about 20 grams of fat a day, which is about 10% of calories from fat.

4. Clean out the kitchen of foods you do not want your family to eat. **Removing temptation** is easier than fighting temptation!

5. Take the shopping list ("for beginners to eating right," chapter 5) and load up on staples. You may want to get some non-stick cookware.

6. Review chapter 14, Menus and Recipes. Pick out 10 and try them! Keep experimenting. Stay open to new foods and combinations.

7. Plan ahead! Read about how to control the Hunger Monster (page 103) and Dining Out fat-free (chapter 6). Think about ways to handle the situations you will find yourself in at a party or a restaurant.

8. Review what a sad diet most Americans eat (SAD page 75).

9. Get to know "beans about beans," page 95. Beans are filling, inexpensive, tasty, and a great source of protein and fiber. Then find out what to do about gas.

10. Eat to your heart's content. You will improve your heart health, cure heartburn, and never worry about hunger. Enjoy!

RATE YOUR DIET

♥ What type of ground beef did you eat last week?

Regular hamburger (30% fat)....................0 point _____

Lean ground beef, lamb (25% fat) ....1 point _____

Extra lean (20% fat), pork, veal ....2 points ____

Ground sirloin or round (10% fat).............3 points ____

Healthy Choice ground beef......................4 points ____

I rarely eat meat, pork, or veal ....5 points ____

♥ What do you eat for breakfast yesterday?
Bacon, eggs, sausage, fried potatoes,
biscuits and gravy, sausage biscuit ....0 point _____
Often skip breakfast ....1 point _____
Egg McMuffin ....3 points ____
Pancakes and syrup ....4 points ____
Cereal, skim milk, orange juice, fruit,
bagel ....5 points ____

♥ What did you eat for lunch yesterday?
Big Mac, Whopper, Fried Fish / Chicken..0 point _____
Often skip lunch ....1 point _____
Lunch meat sandwich................................2 points ____
Lowfat tuna sandwich, 95% lean meat......3 points ____
Peanut butter sandwich or bean burrito,
chicken breast or fish (not fried) ....4 points ____
Baked potato with broccoli or bean soup ..5 points ____

♥ What did you eat <u>with</u> lunch?
French fries, onion rings, chips ....0 point _____
Lowfat chips, lowfat cookies or crackers..3 points ____
Pretzels, rice cakes, fat-free chips ....4 points ____
Fruit or vegetables, salad, vegetable soup.5 points ____

♥ What type of main dish did eat for dinner yesterday?
Ribs, steak, pork chops or similar, pizza ...0 point _____
Hot dogs, hamburgers, fried food..............2 points ____
Ate dinner out-not lowfat ....2 points ____
Fish, chicken breast, other lean meat ....4 points ____
Pasta with marinara sauce, beans, tofu......5 points ____

♥ How often did you eat out last week?

Once or more daily ....0 point _____

Three to four times per week.....................1 point _____

Once or twice a week ....2 points _____

Once or twice a month ....4 points _____

Rarely ....5 points _____

♥ Which meat / protein did you eat yesterday?

(Multiply number of servings by number of points.)

Cheese, eggs, liver heart, brains................0 point _____

High fat cuts of beef, lamb, pork or ham ..0 point _____

Beef round, pork loin, lean ham.................1 point _____

Veal, venison, elk, fish chicken breast.......3 points _____

Beans, legumes, tofu, egg white,

Fat-free cheese, other vegetarian entree ....5 points _____

♥ What kind of milk do you use:

Whole milk (4% fat)...................................0 point _____

Lowfat milk (2% fat).................................1 point _____

1% milk ....3 points _____

1% soy milk...4 points _____

Skim milk (0% fat)....................................5 points _____

♥ Which desserts did you eat yesterday?

Premium ice cream....................................0 point _____

Chocolate, cake, cookies, pie,

regular ice cream, tofutti ....1 point _____

Ice milk, frozen yogurt, sherbet,

lowfat cookies ....3 points _____

Fat-free desserts..4 points _____

Fruit ....5 points _____

Make The Change For A Healthy Heart   **71**

♥ What types of cheese did you eat last week?
Cheddar, Swiss, Jack, Brie,
American, cream cheese.............................0 point _____
Part skim mozzarella, Lappi, light cream
cheese, light cheese, feta, farmer's............2 points _____
Any cottage cheese.....................................4 points _____
Any fat-free cheese....................................5 points _____

♥ How many eggs did you eat last week?
Six or more whole eggs..............................0 point _____
Three to six whole eggs..............................1 point _____
Egg Beaters, Scramblers, Second Nature,
Egg Lights ....4 points _____
Egg whites only- unlimited number..........5 points _____

♥ Which toppings did you use yesterday?
Sour cream, whipping cream, half & half .0 point _____
Light sour cream, Cool Whip Lite.............3 points _____
Non-fat yogurt, non-fat sour cream...........5 points _____

♥ What kind of fat did you cook with yesterday?
Butter, Crisco, lard, bacon grease,
chicken fat ....0 point _____
Stick margarine, ...1 point _____
Tub margarine, olive oil, canola oil...........3 points _____
Light margarine ....4 points _____
None, cooking spray, fat-free spread.........5 points _____

♥ How much added fat did you eat yesterday (i.e. peanut
butter, nuts, margarine, mayo, salad dressing?)
8-10 tsp. or more (average on salad).........0 point _____
6-7 tsp. (average oil for cooking)..............1 point _____

2-3 tsp. (margarine on toast or potato) ......2 points ____

1-2 tsp (average cream in coffee).............3 points ____

I don't add fat...5 points ____

♥ What kind of salad dressing did you use last week?

Real mayo, ...0 point _____

Miracle Whip, Blue Cheese, Russian........1 point _____

Ranch, French, Thousand Island,

Creamy Italian, Lite mayonnaise ....2 points ____

Vinegar and oil, Italian............................3 points ____

Miracle Whip Light, Any light dressing....4 points ____

Fat-free; vinegar; lemon juice; none ....5 points ____

♥ What type of baked goods did you eat yesterday?

Pie, cake with icing, donuts, muffin..........0 point _____

Coffee cake, sweet rolls, french toast........1 point _____

Granola bar, flour tortilla..........................3 points ____

Bread, bagels, corn tortilla ....4 points ____

Oil free bread, low fat bagels, pita bread ..5 points ____

♥ What did you eat for snacks yesterday?

Chocolate, nuts, fatty dessert....................0 point _____

Potato chips, nuts, corn chips ....1 point _____

Buttery crackers, popcorn with fat ....2 points ____

Light popcorn, lowfat crackers or cookies 4 points ____

Pretzels, angel food cake, fat-free cookies,

crackers or chips, sorbet, ...5 points ____

♥ How many pieces of fruit or cups of real fruit juice did you eat yesterday? *Add 1 point per piece:* _____

♥ How many servings of vegetables did you eat yesterday? *Add 1 point per piece:* _____

♥ How many cups of legumes (fat-free refried beans, split peas, navy beans, lentils, meatless chili, etc.) did you eat yesterday? *Add 2 points per serving:* _____

♥ How many servings of each did you have this yesterday?

Wheat germ, brown rice, bulgur, cracked wheat, barley, quinoa, corn, white or sweet potato, whole grain cereal or bread, corn tortillas

Add 2 points per serving: _____

Crackers, popcorn, bagels, pretzels, white bread, flour tortillas, white rice, pasta.

Add 1 point per serving: _____

Score:

100 points or more	→ Excellent lowfat eating.
75 to 100 points	→ On the right track.
50 to 75 points	→ Read this chapter carefully.
Less than 50 points	→ Better get serious about your heart!

Food for Thought:

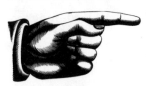

♥ Do you think what you eat can have an effect on your health?

♥ What would encourage you to change what you eat?

♥ Do you read food labels?

♥ What do carbohydrates do in the body?

(See page 52 for more information.)

♥ What is the function of protein (amino acid) in the body?

(See page 50 for more information.)

♥ What is the function of fat (oil) in the diet?

(See page 46 for more information.)

- ♥ What is fiber (roughage)?

   (See page 53 and page 244 for more information.)

- ♥ Do you know any restaurants locally that offer heart healthy meals? When you dine out, is it an opportunity to splurge?

- ♥ Do you frequently dine at "all you can eat" restaurants?

   (See chapter 6 for information on Dining Out fat-free.)

- ♥ If you are "being good" about an eating plan or meal plan, do you frequently feel hungry?

- ♥ What do you want from your food in the next 1 - 3 years?

Please review this quiz with your doctor or dietitian then set a goal:

The first change in my diet I will make is: _____

GOOD LUCK! Now, take what you've learned from this quiz to care for your heart.

SAD (STANDARD AMERICAN DIET)

The Standard American Diet is what we hear on TV and radio, read about, and eat in restaurants (Reference 26):

- ♥ Fat = 40-45%
- ♥ Carbohydrate = 20-30%
- ♥ Protein = 25-40%

Do you recognize the SAD advertisements? The industry spends $40 billion a year to entice you!

- ♥ "Beef, it's what's for dinner" by the American Beef Council.
- ♥ "Milk, it makes a body strong" by the Dairymen's Association.
- ♥ "Pork, the other white meat" by the Pork Producers.

What does it get us?

- ♥ The highest rates of heart disease in the world. In non-Westernized countries, heart disease is much less frequent. As countries take on Western characteristics, the rate of heart disease rises. For example, the Japanese culture was studied. In Japan, heart disease was lowest. Those Japanese moving to Hawaii had intermediate rates. In San Francisco, the heart disease rate among Japanese equalled that of native Americans.
- ♥ Very high rates of certain cancers: colon, breast, prostate. Again, only the USA has these high rates. So called "underdeveloped countries" have much lower rates of these cancers.
- ♥ Food allergies
- ♥ Additives
- ♥ Bacterial contamination of our foods, especially from the sea. Each year, the number of deaths and illness from contamination rises.

AMERICAN HEART ASSOCIATION DIET

The AHA is the standard "therapeutic" diet used by American doctors and dietitians.

- Fat = 30%
- Carbohydrate = 50-60%
- Protein = 10-20%

It is prescribed (usually in less than 1 hour with a Registered Dietitian or in about 10 minutes with a doctor!) It takes an average of 10 hours to adequately learn a low fat meal plan. It has become the "gold standard" for diet therapy, prior to drug prescription.

What does it get us?

Even though it is the "gold standard," every "control group" in studies has steadily declined in health, and has increasing rates of atherosclerosis. The AHA diet is no better than SAD in preventing or reversing heart disease, diabetes, or obesity.

MAKE THE CHANGE MEAL PLAN

Numerous studies have proven the ability of diet to prevent and reverse the process of heart disease. It comes down to this:

- Fat = 10%
- Carbohydrate = 70-80%
- Protein = 10-20%

The Make the Change meal plan contains most all the vitamins, minerals, trace elements, and anti-oxidants we need (except for vitamin E).

What does it get us?

- ♥ Reversal of pre-existing heart disease
- ♥ Improvement and reversal of diabetes
- ♥ Weight loss may be a side effect
- ♥ Improvement of hypertension, the "silent killer"
- ♥ Lowering of cholesterol, even in those with genetically high cholesterol
- ♥ Cancer prevention
- ♥ Prevention of constipation, diverticulosis, hemorrhoids and many other rectal problems
- ♥ Increased energy and vigor
- ♥ Less food allergy, less "spastic colon"
- ♥ No hunger, no "yo-yo" dieting. Most can eat as much as they are used to!

It really is SAD that we are hurting ourselves with our food. Break out of the cage of advertising in which we live. The world is a grand buffet of delicious and exciting foods. Try this plan to eat, drink, and be merry!

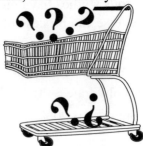

WHAT IS A 10% FAT MEAL PLAN?

The following tables were calculated for average people with average activity levels.

Weight in lbs	Calories	grams of fat
100	1200	13
125	1500	16
150	1800	20
175	2100	23
200	2400	26
225	2700	30
250	3000	33

Table 4. 10% Fat Meal Plan for men

Weight in lbs	Calories	Grams of fat
90	990	11
100	1100	12
125	1375	15
150	1650	18
175	1925	21
200	2200	24
225	2475	27
250	2750	30

Table 5. 10% Fat Meal Plan for women

If you want to reverse heart disease, keep your fat intake at the recommended 10% or less of total calories. This is how we derived table 4 and table 5:

- ♥ **For men:** weight in pounds x 12 = calories a day
- ♥ **For women:** weight in pounds x 11 = calories a day
- ♥ Calories a day x 10% = calories from fat
- ♥ Calories from fat divided by 9 = grams of fat

Make The Change Meal Plan

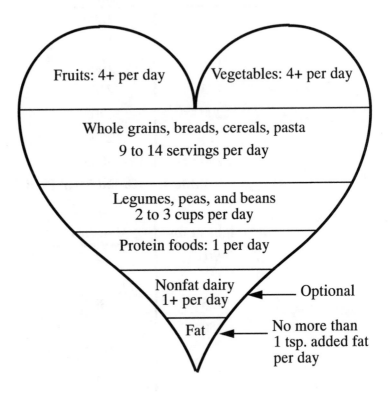

Figure 4. (see chapter 5, page 117 for details)

CHANGING YOUR WAY OF THINKING

WHERE TO BEGIN?

Most of us are very set in our ways when it comes to food. You may have had some experiences that reinforced a typical high-fat diet. Just offer someone "fat-free" food and they may decline (even if the food is delicious). Have you bought something labeled fat-free at the grocery store and been sorely disappointed? You are not alone. Unfortunately, it only takes one bad experience to "turn off" to a whole category of foods.

The good news is that there are many great tasting fat-free foods available. We've done a lot of the legwork and tastework for you and have come up with a list of "Best Fat-Free Foods." See chapter 6.

Cooking fat-free is the same. If you have tried one or two recipes that don't quite meet your standards, you may have said "this fat-free cooking is for the birds" and gone on with your regular way of cooking. However, there are many tricks to fat-free cooking. and we've provided them in a step-by-step way to make it easy to get started.

We only ask one thing--Make the change! Change your way of thinking about food. Leave all those preconceived ideas about vegetarian, fat-free foods behind and open your mind to a way of eating that is delicious, filling and healthy! (It just also happens to be vegetarian and lowfat!) Try to broaden your repertoire of cooking to include other ethnic foods such as Indian, Asian and Middle Eastern. Since these cultures are mostly vegetarian, some of the most wonderful meatless dishes come from those countries.

Eat to live, rather that live to eat.

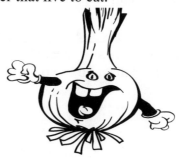

Make The Change For A Healthy Heart

PLANNING AHEAD FOR A FAT-FREE KITCHEN

GETTING STARTED

You've decided to make the change--where do you begin when it comes to food? Just taking the meat off your plate won't be enough--you have to add more of the "good stuff"--pasta, potatoes, vegetables, whole grains, fruit, legumes. Here is a step-by-step plan for arranging your kitchen and your life around your new fat-free but taste-full lifestyle!

Take an inventory of your kitchen. Get rid of all the high-fat foods that you will be tempted to eat. For a list of the foods you'll want to keep on hand, see chapter 5 "Shopping list."

COOKING EQUIPMENT / METHODS

Please take a look at "how" you cook. (If the word "cook" is also a foreign term, turn to convenience foods and dining out in chapter 5 and chapter 6.) Does sauteing or frying come to mind? These are quick cooking methods, no doubt, but let's try to broaden our cooking methods to include fast, convenient and more healthful ways of cooking. Here's a list of equipment for cooking quick, fat-free meals:

Steamer for the stove or microwave. Tupperware makes several types of steamers for microwave. One is a "stack cooker" that allows you to cook 3 dishes at the same time.

Pressure Cooker. If you like to cook beans and grains from scratch, this cooking method will slice the time that you spend in the kitchen.

Crock Pot. Planning ahead by putting your food to cook in a crock pot when you leave for work will have big payoffs. Remember it's at those weak moments when we tend to slip back into old, unhealthier habits.

Stir Fry. Stir-frying in a wok can be done with no added oil (especially if it's non-stick) and is a wonderful way to keep the nutrients in your food.

Food Processor / Vegetable Chopper-slicer. You can prepare veggies more quickly and they will also look more appealing.

Non-stick Saute Pans. Do yourself a favor and buy a new, good quality set of non-stick pans! And don't forget the nylon or plastic utensils made for using with nonstick cookware.

Blender / Food Processor. With a good quality blender, you can make milkshakes, cream soups, creamy sauces and dips. Making a few substitutions will keep those foods flavorful and fat-free.

Deep Freezer. Great for cooking extra and freezing as well as stocking up on foods when on sale.

Breadmaker. Imagine waking up to the smell of homemade cinnamon or hearty sourdough bread every morning! This is possible with a counter-top breadmaker. Fresh bread doesn't need to be slathered in margarine to taste great--it's wonderful all by itself. Remember that on bread isn't something to skimp on, it's something to base your diet on!

CONDIMENTS--SPICE IT UP!

If the spices you use are limited to salt, pepper, garlic salt and cinnamon, then you need to spice up your cooking a bit! When you take out the fat, you will need to add more spices for flavor. Spices add no fat, cholesterol, calories or sodium--what a bargain! Keep in mind that spices lose their taste rather quickly so it's best to keep them for just about six months. Some natural food stores sell spices in bulk so you can buy what you will use in six months.

If buying fresh herbs, wrap in a damp paper towel and place in a zip-lock plastic bag in you refrigerator to keep fresh. Or start your own windowsill herb garden for really fresh herbs!

HERE IS A LIST OF HERBS AND SUGGESTED USES

Allspice: Traditionally used in spice cakes, pumpkin pies, etc., it is a blend of cloves, cinnamon and nutmeg. Try it in sweet potatoes, stews and soups.

Basil: Though Italian cooking comes to mind, basil is actually used in Mexican, Indian, Greek, and Middle Eastern cuisines. Fresh basil goes well in salads, and on pizza and in sauces.

Caraway Seed: Those little seeds found in rye breads also go well in cabbage and noodle dishes.

Cayenne Pepper: In general, just a pinch is wise!

Cinnamon: The spice everyone has--but have you ever thought about using it in green beans or squash or a spicy bean soup?

Cilantro: It is great in making fresh salsas, in salads and cooked in sauces.

Celery Seed: Traditionally used in coleslaw, but also good in soups and stews.

Coriander: The seeds are available whole or in powder form. Try it in curries, sweet dishes and pasta salad.

Cumin: Try it in chilis, soups, beans, and sauces.

Curry: A blend of several herbs. Use it in creamy sauces, traditional curries, in beans and soups.

Cardamom: Try Basmati rice with cardamom seeds. The Basmati rice has a distinctive, nutty flavor and the cardamom seeds give it a wonderful fragrance and taste. Also try in punches and cakes.

Dill Weed: It is great in sauces for vegetables, grains and in salad dressing and dip mixes. This is an easy spice to grow.

Fennel Seed: If you like Italian Sausage, Fennel is one of the predominant spices. Put it in lasagna, vegetarian burgers, and bean loafs to get the same flavor.

Garlic: When in doubt, add garlic! Garlic powder can be used--1/4 teaspoon for each garlic clove. Another shortcut is to buy garlic chopped in a jar. Also garlic has been show to lower cholesterol if you eat it daily.

Ginger: Ginger root is common in Asian and Indian Cooking. It can be used in marinating, in stir fries and in sauces. A shortcut to using it fresh is using a garlic press or grating it. Keep what you don't use in the freezer. Or buy it in a jar. Dried ginger is used in gingerbread, and in sweet vegetables like squash, sweet potatoes and carrots.

Mint: Sure--this is good in iced tea, but it also works well in Indian, Thai and Vietnamese dishes. It often is used as a contrast to hot spices.

Nutmeg: Gives a nice touch to cream sauces and vegetables. Nutmeg is best bought as seeds and freshly ground--similar to using a peppermill.

The Onion Family: Onions of all colors, garlic, chives, shallots and scallions are members. Onion has been shown to lower cholesterol. When you take the fat out, you should add more onion for flavor--experiment with different types!

Saffron: It gives taste to the spanish dish paella. Try it in rice, soups and sauces.

The Mediterranean Family of Spices: Sage, Oregano, Rosemary, Thyme, Savory. These spices are often found together in Italian Seasoning or in the French staple, Herbes de Provence. They are used alone or together in tomato sauces, vegetables, soups, stews and in stuffings.

Tarragon: Wonderful in cream sauces, in salad dressings and marinades.

Turmeric: Another herb that gives a yellow color and a pungent flavor to rice, vegetables and Indian cuisine. It is used in curry.

CUTTING THE SALT

Switching to a plant-based diet automatically cuts a large amount of sodium you would be receiving in processed meats.

Many processed foods contain a significant amount of salt. Make sure to read the label to compare sodium content. Buy no salt added varieties when possible.

- ♥ Canned soups, vegetables, tomatoes and tomato sauce
- ♥ Sauce mixes
- ♥ Teriyaki, soy and stir-fry sauces
- ♥ Frozen dinners and vegetable dishes

Instead of using salt, there are many substitutes:

- ♥ Salt-free seasonings like Mrs. Dash
- ♥ If you just need to "shake some thing"--but don't like the taste of salt substitutes, try Papa Dash - light light salt. (Has 1/4 the sodium of table salt.)
- ♥ Lemon juice--a wonderful flavor enhancer

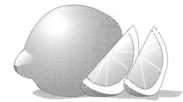

- ♥ Balsamic vinegar
- ♥ Malt vinegar
- ♥ Salt substitutes
- ♥ Garlic powder or fresh garlic
- ♥ More onion or fresh herbs

USING FRESH INGREDIENTS

Using the freshest ingredients will add flavor as well as nutrients to your food. You may want to ask when your grocery gets their shipments of produce, or of specific items. Planning your meals ahead of time (highly recommended) will help. In the summer, take advantage of farmer's markets that are often held several times a week. They guarantee (for the most part) the freshness of the produce. (Even at Farmer's markets, some foods are from out of state, so ask.)

Organically grown produce is also often fresher and healthier, since preservatives aren't used. Fresh herbs as opposed to dried adds more flavor, which is why fine restaurants cook with them. Yes, they are more expensive, but think of how much your grocery bill has gone down now that you aren't buying all those expensive meats! Splurge a little to treat your taste buds. If you really want fresh produce, grow your own! This will also get you outdoors in the summer and you can really enjoy the fruits of your own labor.

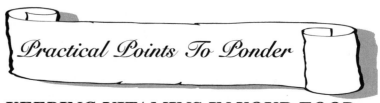

Practical Points To Ponder

KEEPING VITAMINS IN YOUR FOOD

The water soluble vitamins--all the B vitamins and vitamin C are very sensitive to how you treat them. Since they are water soluble, the more liquid you cook them in, the more the vitamin is lost down the drain (unless you save the cooking water for other purposes). Some are also sensitive to light (riboflavin, vitamin C and folic acid) and most are sensitive to heat. More vitamin C is lost if you chop up the food, rather than eat it whole. To keep more vitamins for your good health, follow these tips:

- ♥ Buy fruits and vegetables as you need them. The longer they stay in your refrigerator, the more nutrients are lost.

- ♥ Eating raw fruits and vegetables is best! When cooking, cook in minimal amounts of water or steam. Thaw vegetables (like frozen spinach) instead of cooking them when putting in lasagna or a dip. Frozen vegetables going into salads can also be thawed instead of cooked.

- ♥ Don't wash produce until ready to eat or cook.

- ♥ Keep fruits and vegetables in produce drawer or if cooked, in opaque, airtight container.

- ♥ When possible, buy foods grown locally or from farmer's markets. This helps insure freshness.

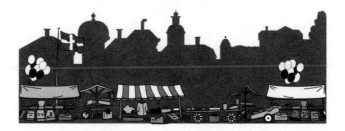

GUIDE TO RECIPE SUBSTITUTION

"Where's The Beef?" and the oil, and the nuts?

... Gone by the wayside with some healthier substitutes listed here to keep on hand.

For Baking:

Instead of	Use
Oil	♥ Applesauce, mashed banana, baby food prunes or other baby food fruit ♥ Mashed sweet vegetable like carrots, sweet potatoes or baby food ♥ Liquid butter buds, fat-free margarine (may not work in all recipes) ♥ Honey
One Whole egg	♥ 1 mashed banana ♥ 2 egg whites or 1/4 cup commercial egg substitute ♥ 2 Tbs. cornstarch or arrowroot ♥ 1/4 cup tofu (blend with wet ingredients before adding to dry)
Butter or margarine in frosting	♥ Marshmallow creme, fat-free cream cheese
Nuts	♥ Grape nuts ♥ Smaller amounts of nuts and chopped more finely. Instead of cooking in the food, sprinkle small amount on top of food.

Table 6.

For Cooking:

Instead of	Use
Oil or margarine for sauteing	♥ Non-stick spray ♥ Fat-free broth ♥ Wine, water, fruit juice, balsamic vinegar ♥ Liquid butter buds
Cream	♥ Evaporated skim milk, plain yogurt, fat-free sour cream ♥ Vegetable purees
Sour cream	♥ Plain nonfat yogurt, fat-free sour cream, pureed tofu ♥ Pureed fat-free cottage cheese plus lemon juice
Cream cheese	♥ Fat-free cream cheese, or pureed fat-free ricotta or cottage cheese
Olives	♥ Capers, Pimientos
Regular cheese	♥ Fat-free cheese--work best when mixed **in** a food like a casserole, or melted in, rather than melted on top ♥ Just a sprinkle of regular cheese--the sharper the flavor, the less you need to add a little zing
Baking chocolate	♥ 3 Tbs. cocoa powder per ounce

Table 7.

AT THE TABLE

On Your Bread:

♥ If you buy fresh bread from a bakery, or make your own, the bread is delicious with **nothing** on it!

Fat-Free Replacements for margarine or butter:

- ♥ Promise Ultra Fat-Free Margarine
- ♥ Roasted garlic (the longer cooked, the milder it gets)
- ♥ Honey or jam / fruit spread
- ♥ Fat-free cream cheese (flavor it by whipping in jam, honey, spices mixes or some fat-free salad dressing mix)
- ♥ Fat-free Boursin Cheese Spread (page 256)

Fillings for Sandwiches:

- ♥ Bean Spread or Guiltless Gourmet Fat-Free Bean Dips
- ♥ Eggless egg salad
- ♥ Fat-free cheese
- ♥ Tossed salad with fat-free cheese and dressing in pita pocket
- ♥ Leftover bean loaf
- ♥ Vegetarian burger (bought frozen and cooked in toaster-oven or microwave)
- ♥ Meatless sloppy joes (page 298)

In place of high fat sandwich spreads:

- ♥ Fat-free mayonnaise
- ♥ Dijon, yellow, german, or gourmet flavored mustard
- ♥ Fat-free "Dijoinaise" (just mix a bit of fat-free mayo or mock mayo with dijon to taste)
- ♥ Salsa
- ♥ Nonfat yogurt
- ♥ Ketchup (sounds a bit funny, but it's really good!)
- ♥ Fat-free honey dijon, italian, or ranch dressing

Other Condiments to Have Available:

- ♥ Low-sodium soy sauce or tamari
- ♥ Worcestershire sauce
- ♥ Salsa
- ♥ Chutney
- ♥ Tabasco or Pick-a-Peppa Sauce
- ♥ Seasoning mix like Mrs. Dash, Seasoned Salt
- ♥ Butter buds or Molly McButter (good for veggies, potatoes)
- ♥ Cajun spice mix

IN PLACE OF MEAT: WHERE'S THE BEEF?

If you like the texture of food you can "sink your teeth into," here are a few substitutes:

For ground beef:

- ♥ **Grains** Bulgur, couscous, rice, oatmeal and millet can be used in soups and chilis and with other vegetables and beans to make "burgers," loafs and other generally meat-containing dishes.
- ♥ **Eggplant** The texture of eggplant also imitates meat. Put it in casseroles, dips and lasagna. Roasted, it is wonderful on pizza, in a sandwich or stuffed in pita bread!
- ♥ **Mushrooms** Have you seen those "Texas sized" mushrooms at your grocery lately? Called Portobello, this variety is big enough for a sandwich. Cook in wine and garlic and have in your sandwich or pasta. Or steam

briefly in the microwave and grill them. Mushrooms can also be used in casseroles, sauces and soups and veggie burgers as a meat substitute.

♥ **Seitan** (wheat gluten): This food is often called "wheat meat." It can be bought frozen in many different ways-- in slices, chicken style, like a roast. It is found already marinated or seasoned in the refrigerated section at large natural food stores. See Faux Fajitas, page 290.

♥ **Tofu** is made from soybeans in a process comparable to making cheese.

The beauty of tofu (and also the reason for its negative reputation) is that it does not have much flavor of its own. It takes on whatever flavor you choose to give it. Therefore it can be used in sizzling Chinese soups, in Southwest chili, as a meat substitute in tacos, as a cheese substitute in lasagne, as a substitute for eggs in "egg salad" or egg foo young. To make tofu have a meatier texture, freeze and thaw and squeeze out excess water. It can be marinated and grilled. Tofu can also be used to make puddings and pies, dips and sauces.

Mori-Nu makes a new lowfat tofu that is vacuum pack-aged. It doesn't need refrigeration so you can stock your pantry. Tofu comes in different textures--which fit for many types of dishes:

♦ Extra firm is good for stir-fry. Firm is good for thick sauces, dips and puddings. Soft / Silken is used for creamy sauces, mock mayonnaise. See recommended resources for more on tofu.

♥ **TVP** Textured Vegetable Protein: This is found in dry granules at the health food store, often in bulk. It works well when substituted for ground beef in soups, chilis, casseroles, and meat loafs.

♥ **Tempeh** is an Indonesian fermented soy product with a texture similar to meat. It can be used in casseroles and other dishes, and also can be used to make "burgers." Tempeh can also be found already marinated in different ways such as Thai, fajita, "burger" patties, etc. at larger health food stores.

♥ **Beans** All beans and peas also make a great meat substitute. The more you learn about beans, the more you'll like them! Checkout the many great varieties. A great source of protein, they taste wonderful too!

Type	Calories in 1/3 cup	Grams of Protein	Grams of Fat	Grams of Carbos
Pinto	75	4.9	0.3	13.6
Kidney	73	4.8	0.3	13.2
Garbanzo	80	4.5	1.1	13.5
Lentils	71	5.2	0.5	12.8
Navy	79	5.2	0.4	14.0
Lima	84	5.0	0.4	15.6
Black	75	4.9	0.3	13.6
Split Pea	77	5.3	0.2	13.9
Soybean	78	6.6	3.4	6.5

Table 8. Beans about beans

INTESTINAL GAS

If you rapidly increase your intake of beans, you may notice a temporary increase in gas. Beans are a great source of fiber, which makes you regular. Intestinal bacteria works to break down sugar in the bean; the result is gas.

Your body rapidly adapts. Soaking, then rinsing beans also helps. The high fiber in foods like beans cures hemorrhoids and cuts your incidence of colon cancer!

BEANO is a product to cut down on gas. It works! It breaks down the nonabsorbable chains of sugar into smaller, absorbable sugars. Besides less gas, the body absorbs more sugar calories. Less fiber is left in the colon.

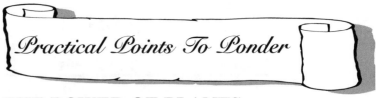

Practical Points To Ponder

THE POWER OF PLANTS

Plant products offer many benefits over animal products-- for what they don't have (saturated fat and cholesterol) and for what they do have (phytochemicals and fiber). For example food made from the soy bean have been shown to enhance health on several ways:

- ♥ Soy protein (TVP, soy milk, tofu, soy beans) have been shown to reduce serum cholesterol (Reference 27)

- ♥ Eating soy protein instead of animal protein seems to affect how much calcium is lost from bone; an important consideration for those concerned with osteoporosis. (Reference 28)

- ♥ In one study, women with the highest soy food consumption had less then 1/2 the risk of breast cancer than those who eat soy rarely. Women with lowest cancer rate eat 2 oz. daily.

♥ Other research showed that eating soy beans or tofu cut the risk of rectal cancer by more than 80%. Just two servings of soy a week seemed to be protective.

Note that soy products contain more fat than some other plant products.

SHORT CUTS TO VEGETARIAN EATING

If in the past, "in a hurry" meant calling out for pizza, going through the drive-thru window for a burger, or just grabbing a donut or chocolate bar, then you need to learn some healthier shortcuts. Here are a few tips that can save you time... and fat!

MAKE EXTRA!

Even if you are just cooking for one or two, make extra and freeze it to use as leftovers. Or, freeze extra portions in microwaveable containers so you can take them for lunch. The following recipes, found in chapter 14, all freeze well:

♥ Stuffed Shells   ♥ Millet Burgers

♥ Vegetarian Chili   ♥ Crustless Quiche

♥ Bean and Rice Burritos ♥ Lentil Soup

Other foods that freeze well include: Pancakes, soups, casseroles, lasagna, muffins, chili, pasta dishes, bean loaves.

USE LEFTOVERS CREATIVELY!

Hardly no one will admit to liking leftovers. However if you just plan ahead a bit, you can use leftovers in a way no one will suspect. Here are a few examples from the recipes in chapter 14:

- ♥ On Monday... Vegetarian chili. On Wednesday... Soft tacos with chili or taco salad with baked tortilla chips
- ♥ On Tuesday... Homemade vegetable soup. On Thursday... Use the leftover vegetables from the soup to go in a curried rice dish
- ♥ On Friday... Mock Egg Foo Young. On Saturday... Oriental burgers with Sweet and Sour Sauce
- ♥ On Sunday... Pinto beans and texmati rice. On Sunday night... Seven layer bean dip with fat-free tortilla chips

BUY CANNED AND CONVENIENCE FOODS

Keep on hand canned beans, fat-free broths, garlic-in-a-jar, soup in a cup, tomatoes, vegetarian chilis, vegetarian burgers and hot dogs (remember that all vegetarian "look alikes" are not necessarily lowfat!) In recipes, the canned foods will save you a lot of time. The convenience foods can be used to make instant meals. See "The Best Fat-Free Foods" on page 122 and "Fifteen-Minute Meals" on page 250.

EASY SAUCES

There are many jarred sauces and sauce mixes that are vegetarian and fat-free. Chinese sweet and sour sauce, ginger and garlic sauce, "Chicken Tonight" and Hain fat-free Brown Gravy Mix are just a few.

KEEP QUICK COOKING GRAINS ON HAND

The old standby is brown rice which can take an hour to cook. Couscous takes 3 minutes. Bulgur and kasha can be cooked in 10-15 minutes or less. Many people prefer the taste of fresh pasta and it cooks in minutes. Grains can also be used as leftovers or cooked in bulk and frozen.

USE SPEEDY COOKING METHODS

Bring out your pressure cooker and use it to cook beans and grains; it will cut your cooking time in half! Don't overlook the microwave for steaming vegetables and grains. A stir-fry meal is quick--especially if you use frozen prepared vegetables and fat-free prepared sauces.

RECIPE MAKE-OVERS

Learn how to take these typical recipes and turn them into a lowfat, vegetarian feast! Here are a few examples

LASAGNA

Serves: 8

Ingredients:

> 1 pound ground beef
>
> 2 cups tomato sauce
>
> 1 Tbs. oil
>
> 1 pound mozzarella cheese, grated, 1/2 cup set aside.
>
> 4 oz. fresh grated parmesan cheese

1 pound cottage cheese

1 onion, chopped

1 garlic clove, chopped

1 package lasagne noodles

Preparation:

1. Saute onion and garlic in oil. Add ground beef. Cook until brown. Drain fat.

2. Cook noodles, adding 1 tsp oil and 1 tsp salt to water.

3. Layer noodles, sauce, ground beef, mozzarella and cottage cheese and parmesan, ending with sauce on top of the last layer of noodles. Sprinkle on 1/2 cup set aside mozzarella.

To modify this recipe:

There are several options for changing this recipe:

Omit 1 pound ground beef... **Save 100 grams of fat!**

Use 1 cup of TVP hydrated in tomato juice or fat-free beef broth, 1-2 packages frozen spinach, cooked with water squeezed out or use sliced eggplant cooked and layered between noodles.

Omit 1 tbs. oil... **Save 14 grams of fat!**

Cook the onion and garlic in broth, wine or water instead.

Instead of 1 pound regular mozzarella cheese... **Use fat - free and save 60 grams of fat!**

Omit 4 oz. fresh grated parmesan cheese... **Reduce to 1 Tbs. and save 28 grams of fat!**

Omit 1 pound regular cottage cheese... **Use fat-free ricotta or cottage cheese and save 20 grams of fat!**

Other ingredients to add...

Add more onion and garlic than called for to spice it up. Add more veggies to the tomato sauce like chopped bell peppers, sun dried tomatoes, fresh herbs, and chopped zucchini. Even if you use bottled tomato sauce, you can still "doctor" it up.

<u>**Total fat saved:**</u> **222 grams or 28 grams per serving!**

CHILI

<u>**Serves**</u>: 8

<u>**Ingredients**</u>:

2 pounds lean ground beef

1 large onion

1 large green pepper

1 28 oz. can tomato sauce

2 Tbs. oil

2 Tbs. chili powder

1 teaspoon salt

15 oz. can kidney beans

1 16 oz. can tomato sauce

8 oz. cheddar cheese, grated

<u>**Preparation**</u>:

1. Using a large pot, saute onion and pepper in oil until tender.

2. Add ground beef and cook, stirring often until brown.
3. Add tomatoes, tomato sauce, seasoning and beans. Simmer slowly for 45 minutes.
4. Serve topped with cheddar cheese and with tortilla chips.

To modify this recipe:

There are several options for changing this recipe:

Omit ground beef... Save 173 grams of fat!

Use TVP rehydrated, or a mix of bulgur and beans and other grains. Some use soy grits to add texture or brown rice. You can also use crumbled firm tofu, chopped seitan or tempeh.

Omit oil... Save 28 grams of fat!

Saute in broth, wine, or tomato juice.

Omit regular Cheddar cheese... Save 72 grams of fat!

Use fat-free cheddar or mozzarella instead.

Omit regular tortilla Chips... Save 72 grams of fat!

Use baked tortilla chips instead. Make your own or try Baked Tostitos.

Ingredients to increase:

Onion, green pepper, and seasonings. You may want to use different varieties and color of beans.

Total fat saved: 345 grams or 43 grams per serving!

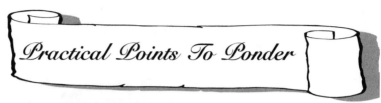

Practical Points To Ponder

CONTROLLING THE HUNGER MONSTER

♥ Eat three meals and two snacks a day. Don't skip breakfast. Instead of letting hunger build all day, snacking prevents overeating in the evening. When you are extremely hungry, anything tastes good and temptation to eat "junk food" is greatest.

♥ Drink lots of water. At no calories, it's a bargain. Drink a glass before eating.

♥ Fat-free goes a long way. At only 4 calories per gram of carbohydrate or protein, you don't have to be afraid of fat-free products in small amounts.

♥ Exercise, at a moderate intensity, helps to suppress the appetite. Exercise daily. Consider taking a short walk when hunger strikes.

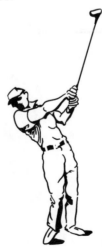

♥ Plan ahead. Have snacks with you. Fruit and cut up vegetables are nutritious, healthy, satisfying, and guilt-free. Keep them available all day.

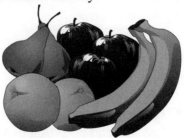

♥ We are more efficient when we snack. Studies on office workers and college students have proven that a mid-afternoon snack prevents the "blahs" and improves productivity and efficiency.

♥ Hunger is a message. Listen to why you eat. If the muscles need energy, feed them. If you are angry, lonely, or depressed; however, you may want to do something about the anger, loneliness and depression. Just because we learned a behavior like overeating doesn't mean it helps us adapt better.

♥ You can't live your life hungry. Learn to feed the hunger, be it physical or emotional.

♥ Get your fill of the other pleasures in life: love, sex, a job well done, runners high, and more.

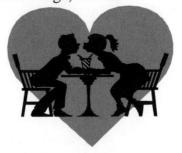

♥ Treat yourself to bite-sized portions. Often a little goes a long way to satisfy hunger.

CHAPTER 5

THE FAT-FREE EATER'S GUIDE TO THE GROCERY STORE

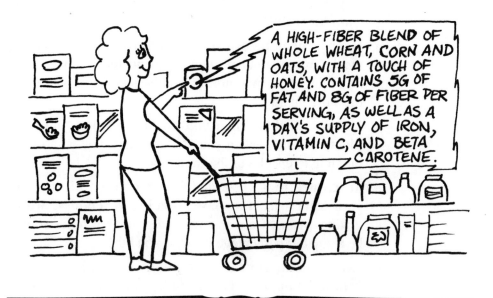

> ## *"Education is not preparation for life; education is life itself."*
>
> *John Dewey*

TEN WAYS TO SHOP SMART

1. **Write out a menu of proposed meals for the week.**
   Make a grocery list according to your menus. You may also want to have a "master list" of foods that you buy weekly or monthly like grains, fruits, vegetables, dried

and canned beans, etc. Keep in mind that many natural foods are also available at mainstream grocery stores and are generally less expensive there.

2. **If you buy from a farmer's market or food co-op, shop there first.**

3. **Have a snack before you go.** Better yet, go right after a meal. The guaranteed way to spend more money (and buy things that may not be health-enhancing) is to go to the store hungry.

4. **Make sure that when you go to the store, you have plenty of time.** When you are in a hurry, you won't have the time to check out the food labels.

5. **To ensure that your diet is top-quality, fill most of your cart with the basics--fruits, vegetables, whole grains, beans.** Convenience and processed foods should be a smaller percentage of what you buy.

6. **Leave home anyone that might be a hindrance to healthy shopping**. This includes children and spouses! On the other hand, it's never too soon (or too late) to teach the benefits of healthy eating. My 4 year-old has already picked up the idea that too much fat isn't good for you. Since many of our "problem" eating habits are learned as children, I'm glad that he is learning healthy eating now.

7. **Expand beyond the foods you usually buy.** Be adventurous. Forego the rice and try quinoa or bulgur. Pass up the crookneck squash and try spaghetti squash. Go tropical! Try mango, papaya, kiwi--not only are they tasty but they are chock full of vitamins.

8. **Read the label** to avoid foods that are high in fat, sodium and other ingredients you may be trying to avoid (or have more of, like fiber).

9. **Always be on the lookout for new fat-free products.** If you hear of a new product but it isn't available at your store, ask the manager to order it for you.

10. **Don't overlook mail-order for some vegetarian and fat-free foods.** *Vegetarian Times Magazine* regularly has listings of vegetarian products by mail.

THE NEW (AND IMPROVED) FOOD LABEL

Just a few years ago, the food label was wreaking havoc on the American public's good intentions of eating healthier. Confusing descriptions of food, claims that had no meaning and serving sizes that were unrealistic made a trip to the grocery store more like a stint on a T.V. quiz show. (Find the **truly** lowfat food and **you** can take it home with you!)

However, all that changed when *The Nutrition Labeling and Education Act of 1990* became law. FDA Commissioner David Kessler describes the changes in food labeling: "The goal is simple: a label the public can understand and count on--that would bring them up-to-date with today's health concerns. It is a goal with 3 objectives: First, to clear up confusion; second, to help us make healthy choices; and third, to encourage product innovation, so that companies are more interested in tinkering with the food in the package, not the words on the label." (Reference 29)

On the page 112 is a sample of the new food label, which you should be a bit familiar with by now:

DEFINING DESCRIPTIONS

Here are the definitions of claims you now see on the label.

Free: Contains either zero, trivial or an amount "physiologically inconsequential" of any of these components: fat, saturated fat, cholesterol, sodium, sugars and calories. "Calorie free" means less than 5 calories per serving. "Sugar-free" and "fat-free" mean less than 0.5 gram per serving. The words "no," "without" and "zero" can be used in place of "free."

Low: This term can be used on foods that could be eaten frequently without exceeding dietary guidelines for one or more of these components: fat, saturated fat, cholesterol, sodium, and calories. Here are some examples:

- ♥ Fat-free: 3 grams or less per serving
- ♥ Low Saturated Fat: 1 gram or less per serving
- ♥ Low Sodium: less than 140 mg. per serving
- ♥ Very Low Sodium: less than 35 mg. per serving
- ♥ Low Cholesterol: Less than 20 mg. per serving
- ♥ Low Calorie: 40 calories or less per serving

High: One serving provides 20% or more of the Daily Value of a nutrient

Good Source: One serving provides 10-19% of Daily Value of a nutrient.

Reduced: The product is nutritionally altered and contains 25% less of a nutrient or calories than the regular or reference product.

Less: This product (nutritionally altered or not) contains 25% or less of a nutrient or of calories than the regular or reference product. "Fewer" can be used instead of "less."

Light: Can mean two things:

1. A nutritionally altered product containing 1/3 fewer calories or 1/2 the fat of the reference food. If the food derives 50% or more of its calories from fat, the reduction must be 50% of the fat.

2. The sodium content of a low-calorie, lowfat food has been reduced by 50%. "Light in sodium" may be used on foods in which the sodium content has been reduced by 50%. This may still contain too much sodium for certain individuals.

More: Contains a nutrient that is at least 10% of the Daily Value more than the reference food.

Percent Fat-Free: Must meet definitions for lowfat or fat-free. The claim must also accurately reflect the amount of fat present in 100 grams (about 3 oz.) of food. If a food contains 5 grams of fat per 100 grams, it must be labeled "95% fat-free."

Healthy: To be labeled healthy, a product has to be lowfat, low in saturated fat, limited in cholesterol and sodium and provide at least 10% of the Daily Value for vitamin A, vitamin C, iron, calcium, protein or fiber. Meal-type products like frozen dinners must provide at least 10% of the Daily Value for two or three nutrients, depending on the type and size of the meal. Sodium limits will be phased in.

KEY CHANGES IN FOOD LABELS

- ♥ Labels contain nutrient information related to **today's** health concerns: fat, saturated fat, cholesterol, dietary fiber.

- ♥ Nutrient information is also shown as a percentage of Daily Value, a reference to show how a food fits into the total diet. Based on 2000 calories per day.

- ♥ New clearly-defined meanings for used for the words "light, low-calorie and high-fiber."

- ♥ Claims about a relationship between a nutrient and a specific disease will be allowed. See list on page 110.

- ♥ Standardized serving sizes which make comparisons between similar products easier.

- ♥ Fruit juices and fruit drinks will have the percentage of fruit juice listed.

- ♥ "Standardized" products such as ice cream and mayonnaise were previously exempt from listing ingredients but will now be required to have an ingredient list.

- ♥ Voluntary nutrition information for many raw foods will be available at point of purchase site.

- ♥ Meat and seafood are **still** not required to have nutrition labeling!

HEALTH CLAIMS ALLOWED ON THE PACKAGE

- ♥ **Saturated fat and cholesterol and coronary artery disease:** Foods using this claim must also meet the definitions for "lowfat," "low saturated fat" and "low cholesterol."

- ♥ **Fat and cancer:** Foods using this claim must also meet the definition for "fat-free."

- ♥ **Calcium and osteoporosis:** Foods using this claim must

The New Food Label at a Glance

The new food label will carry an up-to-date, easier-to-use nutrition information guide, to be required on almost all packaged foods (compared to about 60 percent of products up till now). The guide will serve as a key to help in planning a healthy diet.*

Serving sizes are now more consistent across product lines, stated in both household and metric measures, and reflect the amounts people actually eat.

The **list of nutrients** covers those most important to the health of today's consumers, most of whom need to worry about getting too much of certain items (fat, for example), rather than too few vitamins or minerals, as in the past.

The label of larger packages must now tell the number of calories per gram of fat, carbohydrate, and protein.

Nutrition Facts

Serving Size ¹/₂ cup (114g)
Servings Per Container 4

Amount Per Serving

Calories 90   Calories from Fat 30

                                                    % Daily Value*

Total Fat 3g	**5%**
Saturated Fat 0g	**0%**
Cholesterol 0mg	**0%**
Sodium 300mg	**13%**
Total Carbohydrate 13g	**4%**
Dietary Fiber 3g	**12%**
Sugars 3g	
Protein 3g	

Vitamin A	80%	Vitamin C	60%
Calcium	4%	Iron	4%

* Percent Daily Values are based on a 2,000 calorie diet. Your daily values may be higher or lower depending on your calorie needs:

		Calories	2,000	2,500
Total Fat	Less than		65g	80g
Sat Fat	Less than		20g	25g
Cholesterol	Less than		300mg	300mg
Sodium	Less than		2,400mg	2,400mg
Total Carbohydrate			300g	375g
Fiber			25g	30g

Calories per gram:
Fat 9   •   Carbohydrate 4   •   Protein 4

* This label is only a sample. Exact specifications are in the final rules.
Source: Food and Drug Administration 1993

New title signals that the label contains the newly required information.

Calories from fat are now shown on the label to help consumers meet dietary guidelines that recommend people get no more than 30 percent of their calories from fat.

% Daily Value shows how a food fits into the overall daily diet.

Daily Values are also something new. Some are maximums, as with fat (65 grams or less); others are minimums, as with carbohydrate (300 grams or more). The daily values for a 2,000- and 2,500-calorie diet must be listed on the label of larger packages. Individuals should adjust the values to fit their own calorie intake.

The New Food Label at a Glance

Health Claims: For the first time, food labels will be allowed to carry information about the link between certain nutrients and specific diseases. For such a "health claim" to be made on a package, FDA must first determine that the diet-disease link is supported by scientific evidence. At this time, FDA is allowing seven specific claims about the relationships between:

- fat and cancer risk
- saturated fat and cholesterol and heart disease risk
- calcium and osteoporosis risk
- sodium and hypertension risk
- fruits, vegetables and grains that contain soluble fiber and heart disease risk
- fiber-containing grain products, fruits and vegetables and cancer risk
- fruits and vegetables and cancer risk.

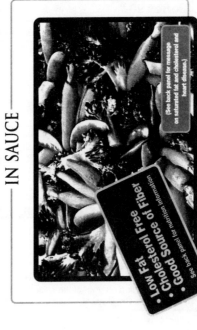

FROZEN MIXED VEGETABLES
— IN SAUCE —

- Low Fat Free
- Cholesterol of Fiber
- Good Source of Fiber

See back panel for nutrition information.

(See back panel for message on saturated fat and cholesterol and heart disease.)

NET WT. 8.9 oz. (252 g)

Ingredients: Broccoli, carrots, green beans, water chestnuts, soybean oil, milk solids, modified cornstarch, salt, spices.

"While many factors affect heart disease, diets low in saturated fat and cholesterol may reduce the risk of this disease."

Source: Food and Drug Administration 1993

Descriptors: While descriptive terms like "low," "good source," and "free" have long been used on food labels, their meaning — and their usefulness in helping consumers plan a healthy diet — have been murky. Now FDA has set specific definitions for these terms, assuring shoppers that they can believe what they read on the package:

- free
- light
- more
- good source
- lean
- extra lean
- high
- low
- reduced
- less

For fish, meat and poultry:

Ingredients still will be listed in descending order by weight, and now the list will be required on almost all foods, even standardized ones like mayonnaise and bread.

Health claim message referred to on the front panel is shown here.

have 20% or more of the Daily Value for calcium (200 mg. per serving), have a calcium content that exceeds the food's content of phosphorous, and contain a form of calcium easily absorbed by the body. See calcium in foods, table 10 on page 156.

- ♥ **Fiber-containing grain products, fruits and vegetables and cancer:** Foods using this claim must meet the definition "fat-free" and must naturally be a "good source" of fiber.

- ♥ **Fruits, vegetables, and grain products that contain fiber and risk of coronary heart disease:** Must meet definition of "fat-free," "low saturated fat" and "low cholesterol," and must naturally contain at least 0.6 grams soluble fiber per serving.

- ♥ **Sodium and hypertension (high blood pressure):** Must meet definition of "low sodium."

- ♥ **Fruits and vegetables and cancer:** Must meet definition for "fat-free" and must naturally be a "good source" of either vitamin A, vitamin C or dietary fiber.

- ♥ **Folic acid and neural tube defects:** Food must be naturally high in folic acid, which has been proven to reduce spina bifida and other birth defects of the spinal canal.

EXCEPTIONS TO THE RULES:

As is true with most rules, there are exceptions:

- ♥ Fat-free milk can be called "lowfat" even though it doesn't meet the lowfat definition of 3 grams of fat per serving. Lowfat milk can contain up to 5 grams of fat per serving. Only buy skim milk!

- ♥ Food produced by small companies is exempt--based on the number of employees and number of units produced in one year.

- ♥ Foods served for immediate consumption--as on an airplane or in a restaurant, are exempt.

- ♥ Ready to eat food that is not for immediate consumption--such as from a grocery deli or bakery are exempt.

- ♥ Plain coffee, tea, spices and other foods which contain no significant amount of nutrients are exempt.

- ♥ The term "light" can still be used to describe texture and color as in "light brown sugar" or "light and fluffy."

- ♥ Food in small packages, like life savers, are not required to carry a food label. However, the phone number or address of the company must be listed so consumers can get nutrition information.

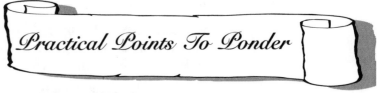

Practical Points To Ponder

LABEL LOGIC

An easy way to put the new food label to work for you:

- ♥ **Check out the serving size.** All the information on the label is based on that serving size. If the serving size is 1/2 cup, but you'd typically eat one cup, you need to multiply all the nutrient information by two.

- ♥ **Look at the fat grams.** Ignore all the percentages for fat, saturated fat, cholesterol etc. Remember those percentages are based on a 30% fat, 2000 calorie diet or 65 grams total fat. Your fat budget is about 20 grams, so you should just compare the total fat grams to your goal for the day. A good rule of thumb is to aim for 5 grams of fat per meal with the extra 5 grams of fat dispersed between snacks throughout the day. With that in mind, if a food is to be the main dish or entree, 3-4 grams of fat would be acceptable. However if the food is just an accompaniment or side dish, look for foods with to 0-2 grams of fat.

❤ **Look at the saturated fat grams.** All fats are a mixture of polyunsaturated, monounsaturated and saturated. See figure 1 on page 47 to find out the typical amount of saturated fats in different oils and fat. By choosing the food with the lowest amount of fat you will probably be getting the food with the least amount of saturated fat.

❤ **Will extra fat be needed in the preparation of this food?** Many times, the label lists fat for the packaged mix, but not as prepared. Also keep in mind that you should be able to omit most oil or use the substitutions for fat listed on page 89.

❤ **Look at other nutrients on the label:** sodium, fiber and vitamins. Vitamins are given in percentages of Reference Daily Intakes or RDIs. The RDIs are the same as the US RDA's, and are based on the Recommended Dietary Allowances created in 1968 for food labeling. These levels may not reflect current thinking about dietary needs. Your fiber goal is 25-30 grams per day--an easy goal with the Make the Change Program. Sodium intake should be below 2,400 mg. per day.

❤ **Remember that just because a product is vegetarian, it isn't necessarily lowfat!** Peanut butter is made from a plant but a majority of its calories come from fat!

❤ **There may not be a nutrition label.** You will find a larger number of products made by small companies-- they aren't required to have food labels. Your next strategy is to look at the ingredient list, which lists ingredients in descending order by weight. Oil should be at the bottom of the list and definitely not in the first half of ingredients. You can also check the ingredient list to find the type of fat used in the product.

♥ **Remember that "fat-free" doesn't mean "calorie free."** Fat-free foods can be delicious--to the point that it may be hard to stop eating them! A friend of ours can eat a whole box of Snackwell cookies! It isn't a problem for him because he burns the calories off--but it could be for more sedentary folk!

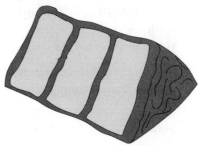

QUESTIONS YOU MAY HAVE

♥ **When I looked at a label, the food was labeled "Fat-Free" and there was 0 gram of fat but 4 calories from fat. How can the food be labeled fat-free even though there are calories from fat?** The grams of fat listed are rounded off. Technically, if a product has 0.5 gram of fat or less, it can be called "fat-free." The grams of fat are rounded up or down, so to figure out exactly how much fat is in the product, divide the calories from fat by nine.

♥ **What should I think about a product that has 6% Daily Value for fat?** We suggest you ignore the percent Daily Value for fat, saturated fat and cholesterol. Those numbers are based on a 2,000 calorie meal plan that contains 30% fat. The Make the Change Meal Plan strives for 10% fat and may be higher or lower in calories. See page 78 for your suggested daily calories based on weight and sex.

Make The Change Meal Plan

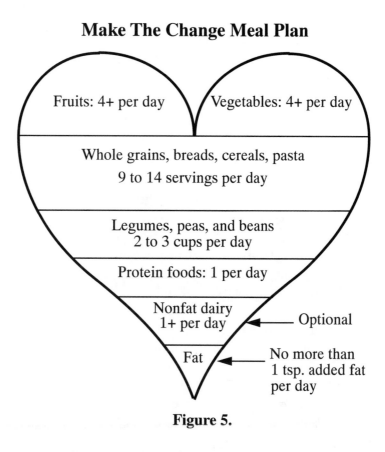

Figure 5.

HEALTHY FOODS SHOPPING LIST FOR EATING RIGHT

This is a basic list to get you headed in the right direction. This may not be all you want to eat, but all these foods are good to your heart, and help to prevent cancer. They are all very low in fat. You may notice unexpected weight loss if you stick to these foods only.

Whole grains:

Amaranth	Barley	Buckwheat
Bulgur	Corn	Millet
Oats	Popcorn	Quinoa
Rice	Rye	Sorghum
Triticale	Wheat berries	Wheat

Vegetables:

Arugula (a green)	Asparagus	Bamboo shoots
Beets	Broccoli	Brussels sprouts
Burdock	Cabbage	Carrots
Cauliflower	Celery	Celery root
Chicory	Chili peppers	Cocozelle
Collard greens	Cucumbers	Daikon
Eggplant	Endive	Escarole
Jerusalem artichoke	Jicama	Kale
Leeks	Lettuce	Mushrooms
Mustard greens	Okra	Onions
Radishes	Rutabagas	Scallions
Spinach	Sprouts	Squash
Sweet potato	Swiss chard	Taro
Turban squash	Turnips	Water chestnuts
Watercress	White potato	Yams
Zucchini		

Fruits:

Apple	Apricots	Banana
Blackberries	Blueberries	Cantaloupe
Carambola	Casaba melon	Cherimoya
Cherries	Cranberries	Currants
Dates	Figs	Guava
Grapefruit	Grapes	Honeydew melon
Kiwifruit	Kumquat	Lemon
Lichee	Limes	Loganberries

Loquat	Mango	Nectarine
Orange	Papaya	Passion fruit
Peach	Pear	Persimmon
Pineapple	Plantain	Plum
Pomegranate	Prune	Pummelo
Quince	Raisins	Raspberries
Strawberries	Tangelo	Tangerine
Tomato	Watermelon	

Legumes:

Azuki beans	Black beans	Black eyed peas
Chick peas	Fava beans	Garbanzo beans
Green peas	Kidney beans	Lentils
Lima beans	Mung beans	Navy Beans
Pinto beans	Split peas	White beans

Protein foods:

| Egg whites | Lowfat Soy milk | Nonfat dairy products |
| Seitan | Tempeh | Tofu |

Beverages:

| Fruit juice | Herbal teas | Vegetable juices |
| Seltzer | Skim milk | Water |

Desserts and snacks:

Ice cream substitutes: sorbet, fat-free yogurt, popsicles

Fat-free Cakes and Cookies: like Entenman's, Snack Wells, Health Garden, Fat-Free Fig Bars (Nabisco and Mother's) See page 123 for The Best Fat-Free Foods.

Try different combinations and additions to give more variety. Don't forget that the color, amount, presentation and smell of your food will enhance your enjoyment.

Make The Change For A Healthy Heart

INGREDIENT GUIDE TO VEGETARIAN EATING

Miso, Quinoa, Seitan: A new language? No, just some of the new foods you might want to try on a health enhancing eating plan! Here is a guide to ingredients which may be new and different to you.

Buckwheat / kasha: It is available as buckwheat flour, groats or when groats are toasted is called kasha. You may see kasha as a type of breakfast cereal in health food stores. Kasha has a hearty flavor and cooks rather quickly.

Bulgur: Use it in place of rice. It cooks quickly--with some types you just need to pour boiling water and let it set. Bulgur is higher in fiber than brown rice and is the basis for the dish "tabouleh."

Capers: are small buds that are usually pickled. They are great in salads, sauces and are a good substitute for olives on a vegetarian pizza.

Chick peas: Are also called garbanzo beans and you will frequently find them on salad bars. They make wonderful sandwich spreads, dips, and vegetarian burgers. They are high in protein and fiber. See page 257 for "Cajun garbanzo nuts."

Couscous: Traditionally made from crushed wheat, the couscous found in the grocery is closer to a tiny pasta and is quick cooking.

Lentils: are a quick cooking legume that are very versatile. Red lentils cook even more quickly than dry lentils since they are split in half when dried. They don't need to be soaked before cooking. Lentils are high in protein, folacin, iron, zinc, thiamin and fiber.

Millet: is a small seed that is mild flavored and is similar to rice in texture and flavor. Use it in place of rice or in a "Millet Burger" page 293.

Miso: is a naturally aged soybean paste used for adding flavor to soups, sauces, etc. Three types of miso found in the U.S. are red (made from rice and soybeans), hatcho (made from soybeans) and barley (made from barley and soybeans).

Nutritional Yeast: is a common flavoring in vegetarian cooking. It is available in flakes or powder form and gives food a "cheesy" taste. Try it in soups, stews, sauces or on popcorn. It is often a good source of vitamin B_{12}. Check the label. Don't confuse nutritional yeast with dry active yeast or brewers yeast, which both taste terrible!

Pine Nuts: Also called pinola. Like other nuts, they are high in fat, so use sparingly. Try them roasted on salads.

Quinoa: is a high protein grain with a texture similar to barley. Rinse before cooking and use in place of rice, or in salads with beans and vegetables.

Sea Vegetables: Examples are nori, dulse, kombu, wakame and arame. Agar agar is a substitute for gelatin.

Sesame Oil: is a strong tasting oil used in Asian cooking. Because the flavor is so concentrated, **just a few drops** imparts a wonderful flavor to your cooking.

Soy Sauce: An aged product made from soy beans and often wheat. Tamari is similar to soy sauce but it is made with little or no wheat. Soy sauce is very high in sodium, although lower sodium versions are available. Kikkoman Lite Soy Sauce contains 100 mg. sodium in 1/2 a teaspoon.

STORING WHOLE FOODS

Hopefully, you are changing your buying habits to include more "whole" foods such as whole grains and beans. Here are a few tips for storing them to keep their quality. Keep the following **in the refrigerator**: Whole grain flour, nuts, seeds and nut butters, tofu, whole grain breads and baked goods.

THE BEST FAT-FREE FOODS

Going through all the fat-free products now available could take months! We put together several panels of tasters including cookbook authors, wellness specialists, Preventive Health Institute participants, weight loss class participants and registered dietitians to find out which foods tasted best. To taste all the fat-free foods available would be impossible; this list will give you a start! As this book is going to print, there are already plenty of new fat-free foods going on the market, so just because a food isn't listed here doesn't mean it's not good!

We also found that in some cases there was a wide variety of reactions to the food, depending on personal preferences. When talking to clients and friends, it seems like the main brand names keep popping up: Healthy Choice, Entenmann's and Snackwell. Also, don't overlook the store brands (such as Safeway Enlighten) who are introducing new salad dressings, soup in a cup, etc.

All the foods listed are either fat-free or very lowfat. Here are the results:

Best crackers:

- ♥ Snackwell: Cracked Pepper Crackers / Classic Golden
- ♥ Premium Fat-Free Saltine Crackers

Best snack foods:

- ♥ Tostito's Baked Tortilla Chips
- ♥ Rold Gold Fat-Free Pretzels
- ♥ Louise's Maui Onion Potato Chips

Best canned soups / chili's:

- ♥ Healthy Choice Country Vegetable / Garden Vegetable
- ♥ Progresso Lentil Soup / Black Bean Soup
- ♥ Health Valley Tomato Vegetable Soup
- ♥ Health Valley Vegetarian Chili's (there are several levels of spiciness)

Best salad dressings:

There was a wide variation in scores for dressings, depending on a person's preference for sweet, tangy, etc.

- ♥ Hidden Valley: Fat-Free Ranch / Italian Parmesan
- ♥ Kraft Free: Thousand Island / Catalina

Best soup in a cup:

- ♥ Spice Hunter Fettucini and Broccoli
- ♥ Knorr Black Bean
- ♥ Fantastic Foods: Jumpin' Black Bean / Bombay Curry Rice And Beans

Best vegetarian burgers:

- ♥ Natural Touch Vegetarian Burgers
- ♥ Garden Chef Garden Mexi Burgers

Best pasta sauce:

- ♥ Campbell's Garlic
- ♥ Healthy Choice Traditional

Best cookies:

- ♥ Snackwell's: Fudge Cookie Cakes / Devil's Food Cookie Cakes / Reduced Fat Chocolate Chip Cookies
- ♥ Mother's and Fig Newton Fat-Free Fig Bars

Best "ice cream" product:

We only heard good things about any of Healthy Choice Premium Lowfat Ice Cream.

- ♥ Healthy Choice Lowfat Ice Cream: Mint Chocolate Chip / Malt Caramel Corn
- ♥ Cascadian Farm Strawberry Sorbet

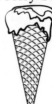

QUESTIONS YOU MAY HAVE ABOUT FAT-FREE FOOD

♥ **Why is sugar often the first ingredient listed in fat-free cookies and cakes?**

When the fat is taken out, something must be added to keep the product moist. This is often sugar. If you are trying to stay away from sugar, look for Health Valley products, which are sweetened with fruit, or try making your own.

♥ **What are all those funny sounding ingredients in fat-free salad dressings and cheeses?**

When you take out the fat in those products, something must be added to give the texture and mouthfeel of fat. Though they sound like exotic chemicals, most are from plants and trees. Here are a few common ingredients:

♦ **Cellulose gum:** Added to cheese to keep it soft and smooth. Modified form of a substance found in plants.

♦ **Xanthum gum:** One of many gums that are added to cheese and salad dressing to thicken them. Made from corn syrup. Other gums are carob bean gum (from the locust tree) and gum acacia (from the acacia tree).

♦ **Carageenan:** Used in salad dressings and even lowfat hamburger beef as a thickener and fat substitute. It is made from seaweed.

♥ **Can you eat too many fat-free products?**

Make sure you get your daily fill of grains, beans, fruits and vegetables before eating fat-free products. Fat-free desserts are highly processed and loaded with sugar; easy to eat, but the calories do add up!

PACKING YOUR SNACK STASH

Good News! "Snack" is no longer a four-letter word! On a lowfat eating plan, snacking is essential--you just need to make sure your snacks are healthy. Keep snacks with you at work and in the car to avoid having to stop somewhere and be tempted by high fat foods.

Crunchy:

- ♥ Unsalted pretzels, crackers, baked chips or tortilla chips
- ♥ Popcorn cakes
- ♥ Rice cakes (Sweetened or unsweetened)
- ♥ Homemade trail mix
- ♥ Fresh apple
- ♥ Fat-free granola or granola bar
- ♥ Fresh vegies: cucumber, tomato, celery, ...

Soft / Sweet:

- ♥ Fresh fruits: pear, banana, mango, pineapple, ...
- ♥ Raisins, dried apricots, prunes
- ♥ Fat-free pudding
- ♥ Jello
- ♥ Fat-free cakes (like Entemann's)
- ♥ Fat-free yogurt
- ♥ Leftover pancakes with syrup (warm in toaster)
- ♥ Fat-free muffin
- ♥ Fat-free frozen yogurt with Hershey's chocolate syrup

Warm:

- ♥ Soups: vegetable soup, bean soup, consomme
- ♥ Fat-free cheese dip / bean dip (Guiltless Gourmet)
- ♥ Baked potato with salsa

CHAPTER 6

EATING AWAY FROM HOME

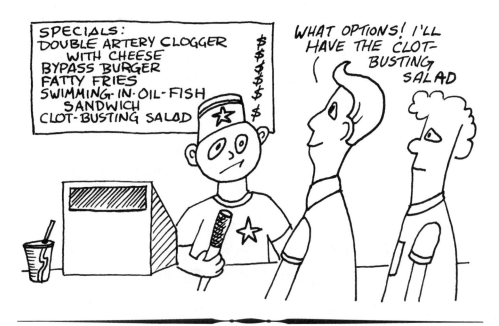

"Home is where the heart is."

FAST FOOD

We probably don't need to tell you--we live in a fast-paced world. However, the hectic pace of our lives shouldn't be allowed to destroy our health! Just in case you are waiting for your life to slow down before starting a new way of eating--be realistic! You'll probably never find that "perfect" time where there is a lull in your schedule... Unless it's that quiet time in the hospital after another heart attack!

There's a positive trend growing among the fast food giants. Taco Bell recently introduced a "Border Lite" menu using reduced fat meats and fat-free sour cream and reduced fat/fat-free cheeses. A family style restaurant in Colorado Springs is offering fat-free cheeses as an option. Who knows? McDonald's next new menu item may be a vegetarian burger! Already, there are healthy options at many fast food restaurants. You needn't give up on "grab and go" type meals--just choose more carefully and stay away from places that don't offer a healthy choice. Also, let restaurants know that you are avoiding them until they have a lowfat vegetarian option on the menu.

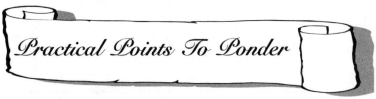

Practical Points To Ponder

FAST FOOD TIPS

- ♥ Most fast-food restaurants have salads or salad bars but don't carry fat-free dressing--bring your own.

- ♥ Vegetarian items such as refried beans will still have added fat. Ask if lard is used and, if so, avoid them!

- ♥ If a food is called "vegetarian" don't order it automatically. Those foods often have more added fat than other foods. The Veggie Cheese Melt at Denny's has 39 grams of fat!

- ♥ Since it is still difficult to make a complete meal at most fast food restaurants, bring some fruit and other snacks to fill in.

♥ Keep in mind that the choices at many fast food outlets are very limited--they can feed you enough to get by to your next snack but may not be a complete meal.

GOOD CHOICES

Breakfast:

🍎 Pancakes with syrup (skip the butter)

🍎 Fat-free muffins (McDonald's), english muffin (ask for it dry) with jam (McDonald's)

🍎 Bagel or toast with jam or honey

🍎 Cereal and skim milk

🍎 Egg Beaters--good with mushrooms, onions, peppers (prepared without added fat)

Lunch and Dinner:

🍎 Bean Burrito or Tostada without cheese or fat-free cheese (ask for lettuce and tomato)

🍎 Tossed salad or salad bar

🍎 Baked potato (Wendy's, Arby's and Hardee's)

🍎 Meatless burger (ask them to leave off the meat and add more tomato, lettuce, onion, pickle, and mustard)

🍎 Vegetable soups (Arby's)

🍎 A meal of side dishes--often served at chicken, BBQ and fish restaurants: Rice, baked beans, green beans, carrots, mashed potatoes, salad, peas, corn

🍎 Noodles or rice bowl--served at many fast food restaurants in California and Hawaii

Desserts:

- ❤ Fat-free frozen yogurt (Dairy Queen, TCBY, I Can't Believe It's Not Yogurt and many others)
- ❤ Sorbet and ice (Baskin Robbins, Haagen Daaz and other ice cream stores)

Follow Frank for lunch:

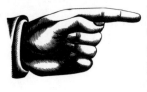 Frank Barry usually fits in a workout at the "Y" during lunch but still has time to fit in a quick healthy lunch. He goes to Wendy's and gets the Baked Potato Bar and tops the potato with broccoli and salsa.

Here are some specific fast food menus. **All menus have eight grams of fat or less.**

- ❤ *Arby's*
    - ❤ Plain baked potato with au jus
    - ❤ Lumberjack mixed vegetable soup
    - ❤ Side salad with lite Italian dressing
- ❤ *Au Bon Pain* (has many good choices!)
    - ❤ Split pea soup and hearth roll
    - ❤ Vegetarian lentil soup and petit pain
    - ❤ Vegetarian chili and onion bagel

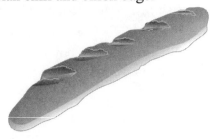

♥ *Boston Market* (Formerly Boston Chicken)
  - Steamed vegetables
  - New potatoes
  - Fruit salad
♥ *Carl's Jr.*
  - Baked potato lite with salsa; hold the butter
  - Side salad
  - Orange Juice
♥ *Captain D's*
  - White beans
  - Seasoned green beans
  - Rice
  - Dinner salad with low calorie italian dressing
  - Bread sticks (up to 4, no added butter or salt)
♥ *El Pollo Loco*
  - Vegetarian burrito
  - Side salad with salsa
  - Corn tortilla
♥ *Grandy's*
  - Baked beans
  - Green beans
  - Seasoned rice or corn
♥ *KFC*
  - Red beans and rice
  - Garden rice
  - Green beans
  - Mean greens

♥ *Kenny Rogers Roasters*
  - ◉ Corn on the cob
  - ◉ Steamed vegetables
  - ◉ Honey baked beans
  - ◉ Side salad

♥ *Long John Silver's*
  - ◉ Rice pilaf
  - ◉ Side salad with your own fat-free dressing
  - ◉ Green beans
  - ◉ Baked potato

♥ *Macheezmo Mouse* (caters to the health conscious)
  - ◉ Vegetarian burrito dinner and vegetables
  - ◉ Vegetarian taco dinner and mixed greens

♥ *Pizza*
  - ◉ 4 slices pizza with sauce, bell peppers, mushrooms, onions, tomato and pineapple (no cheese & ask that no extra oil be brushed on)
  - ◉ Side salad with your own fat-free dressing

♥ *Roy Rogers*
  - ◉ Plain baked potato with gravy
  - ◉ Side salad
  - ◉ Baked beans

♥ *Taco Bell*
  - ◉ Border lite bean burrito (ask for fat-free cheese)

♥ *Wendy's*
  - ◉ Baked potato bar with steamed broccoli, tomato and salsa
  - ◉ Side salad with veggies, beans and fresh fruit

AT THE SALAD BAR

Tips:

♥ If you fill your plate up with only "rabbit food" you will be hungry an hour later! You also need to add some starchy foods like beans and corn and have some bread or crackers and fruit.

♥ If you use "regular" salad dressing, you will turn a fat-free meal into a high-fat disaster. Bring your own fat-free, use vinegar or lemon or a lowfat dressing.

Depending on the restaurant, a salad bar can be a great place to eat a lowfat meatless meal.

Here's how the typical offerings on the salad bar rate.

Good Choices:

● Lettuce, spinach, radishes

● Broccoli, tomatoes, carrots, celery, corn

● Pasta salad (Most are surprisingly low in fat!)

● Three bean salad, kidney beans, garbanzo beans

● Any other bean mixtures or grain mixtures

● Canned or fresh fruits

● Jello salad

Poor Choices:

● Macaroni salad, potato salad

● Fried vegetables, fried chinese noodles

● Cheese, ham

● Sunflower seeds and nuts (unless you use very little)

- Olives (unless you use very little)
- Pudding, mousse

DINING OUT, FAT-FREE

OK. So now you understand the importance of fat-free dining to your health and well-being. You cook and eat fat-free at home. But what about dining out? Will you be frustrated, embarrassed, or tempted? The following is a story which offers some suggestions to help you stay on course.

My brother-in-law Dave wanted to celebrate a family reunion. Being a very dedicated vegetarian, he knew the rest of the family members might feel deprived at a vegetarian only restaurant. But Dave was resourceful. Planning ahead, he was able to find his favorite food in a beautiful downtown San Francisco restaurant that also specialized in seafood.

The reunion came off without a hitch. Three generations ate to their heart's content. Those with special dietary needs were accommodated, and the others enjoyed the fresh seafood. Everyone left satisfied because the ambiance, presentation, color, taste and amount were attended to. A great meal!

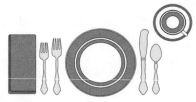

TO AVOID FRUSTRATION

If eating at a friend's home, explain your program ahead of time. Your friends will understand. Often, if you blame "this crazy meal plan" on your doctor (and I encourage you to, at least initially) an alternative can be planned. Better yet, offer to bring a delicious fat-free entree yourself!

Call ahead to the restaurant when eating out. Remember it's your money to spend wherever you choose. Most finer establishments will be eager to cater to your needs. Be very precise about your needs, however, and don't assume they know how to cook fat-free.

TO AVOID EMBARRASSMENT

Let everyone in your party know you are eating fat-free. This will generate many interesting conversations about your choice, and is a good opportunity to EDUCATE your friends and be the center of conversation. However, make it clear this is your personal decision, and that your friends may eat whatever they choose.

At restaurants, check that menu choices that fit your eating style are offered. If not, call ahead and request a fat-free meal. If they cannot or will not provide a fat-free meal, suggest an alternate (better) restaurant to your friends.

TO AVOID TEMPTATION

Pre-eat. That's right. If you know you will succumb, eat a meal or a snack at home. It will be easier to stick to the vegetables and bread if you are already full. But to endear yourself to the host, offer to bring a fat-free plate to the party. Not only will you help the hosts, but you will help yourself.

At restaurants, speak to the waiter immediately. Ask that the high-fat hors d'oeuvres and desserts not be placed in front of you. If you already have scanned the menu, order even before being seated. Let the waiter know you have special requirements and they usually go out of their way to please.

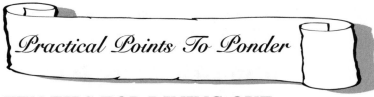

Practical Points To Ponder

TEN TIPS FOR DINING OUT

1. Call ahead to ask if the restaurant you are planning to visit has any vegetarian foods or can specially cook something up for you. Most nicer restaurants can easily do this.

2. When you are seated, ask the hostess that your server not bring the customary chips, crackers, biscuits or other high-fat, pre-meal snacks. Also ask that they leave off the butter or margarine from the bread basket.

3. Have in mind what you will order when you get there. This will keep you from looking at the menu and being tempted.

4. If there is a shadow of a doubt about how a food is prepared or what ingredients it contains, ask! You may need to ask for a manager to get the correct information.

5. Ask in advance that all sauces, margarine, and sour cream be left off or served on the side. Also request that your toast or vegetables not be brushed with any margarine, oil or butter.

6. If you are unhappy with the way the food is prepared-- I.E. fried or a layer of oil on top--SEND IT BACK! You are paying for your meal, and you should be happy with it.

7. Keep in mind that you are almost always getting more fat than you think you're getting when you eat out! Budget for it.

8. Bring with you anything that will help stay on track--fat-free dressing, package of butter buds, salt-free seasoning.

9. If you are ordering an alcoholic drink for your meal, have it with your meal, not before. Drinking on an empty stomach can increase your appetite and make it tougher to pass up the chips, bread, etc.

10. Most restaurants offer a dinner or garden salad. However, many add cheese, croutons, olives, nuts, etc. that will increase it's fat content. Ask about salad ingredients!

<u>Food for Thought:</u>

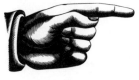

ENJOY YOUR DINING EXPERIENCE, in presentation, amount, color and taste. Don't forget the warm ambiance of friendly conversation and camaraderie! You will most likely enjoy your new eating style more than the old one, and I guarantee you will feel better when you leave the table.

COMMON RESTAURANT FOODS THAT ARE FAT-FREE OR LOWFAT

MEXICAN

Tips:

1. Call ahead to see if the restaurant has any vegetables they can steam or grill for you, such as squash. If so, you can make your own vegetarian fajita out of it--skip the cheese.

2. Ask if the refried beans and rice are cooked with oil or lard. If so, find a restaurant that cooks with your health in mind. Ask if you can bring your own baked tortilla chips.

3. Ask the waitress to forego bringing the chips.

Suggested Menu:

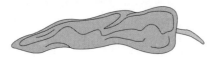

- Steamed vegetables (if available) with salsa or fat-free vinaigrette (bring your own)
- Bean tostada (ask if the corn tortilla can be baked instead of fried) topped with lettuce, tomato, peppers and salsa
- Mexican rice (if cooked without oil)
- Baked sopapilla with honey (ask them to bake instead of fry the sopapilla)

Other Good Choices:

- ❤ Bean or vegetable stuffed enchilada
- ❤ Steamed corn or flour tortillas
- ❤ Bean tacos

Fat-free Accompaniments: Salsa, lettuce and tomato, tabasco

CHINESE

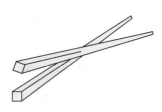

Tips:

- ♥ Call ahead and find out if they can cook your meal without added oil.
- ♥ Find out what foods on the menu are fat-free.
- ♥ If ordering a full meal that includes a high-fat egg roll or fried rice, ask what can be substituted for it.
- ♥ Dim Sum is served on weekends at many Chinese restaurants. Carts are passed from table to table with small portions of many different foods. The ability to see a food before you eat it makes this a good choice.
- ♥ Tofu or bean curd is common in Asian cooking and can probably be substituted in any dish containing meat. Ask them to steam it instead of frying it.
- ♥ If you order noodles, make sure the noodles are soft and not fried or tossed with oil.

Make The Change For A Healthy Heart **139**

Suggested Menus:

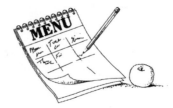

- Hot and sour soup
- Mixed vegetables with garlic sauce
- Steamed rice

- Won ton soup
- Vegetable Lo Mein (ask that it be prepared without oil)

- Steamed dumplings
- Bean curd with vegetables
- Steamed rice
- Hot tea and fortune cookie

Lowfat Accompaniments: Chinese mustard, plum sauce, soy sauce (high sodium)

ITALIAN

Tips:

- Call ahead and find out if steamed vegetable and other lowfat foods are available. Ask if any dishes such as manicotti can be prepared with just vegetables.
- Bring your own fat-free salad dressing and butter buds for pasta.
- Ask which sauces are meatless and cheeseless.
- Ask for plain Italian bread instead of garlic bread. If bread sticks are served ask that they not brush them with butter or add cheese.

<u>Suggested menus:</u>

- Tossed Salad with red wine vinegar (or bring your own fat-free dressing)
- Baked ziti with marinara sauce
- Italian bread (no butter)
- Rasberry sorbet

- Tossed salad with lemon wedge or fat-free dressing
- Spaghetti with marinara sauce
- Steamed vegetables
- Cappucino with Amaretto

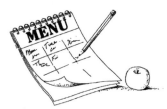

- Lentil soup
- Pasta primavera without added fat
- Fresh fruit

- Vegetable soup
- Spinach stuffed shells with marinara sauce (ask if they can leave out the cheese or use just a little)

<u>Light lunch at Olive Garden:</u>

- Pasta E Fagioli Soup
- Tossed salad (ask that the dressing be not added to the salad)
- Bread sticks (no oil or butter brushed on)

INDIAN

Indian food is mostly vegetarian but it is far from being fat-free! With some education, some help from your waiter and a bit of creativity in the kitchen, Indian food can be lowfat!

Suggested Menus:

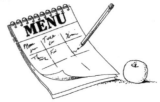

- Green salad with chutney
- Dahl with basmati rice
- Curried vegetables
- Chapatti bread
- Peppermint tea

- Dholkas (steamed rice and bean cakes)
- Onion nan (roasted bread stuffed with onions and spices)
- Kachumbar salad (cucumber and tomato salad)

- Khasta rosti (roasted bread)
- Dosa (thin pancakes stuffed with potatoes)
- Raita (yogurt and vegetables)
- Mazzo mango drink

The above information was compiled from *Simple, lowfat and Vegetarian* by Suzanne Havala M.S. R.D. © 1994, Vegetarian Resource Group.

AT THE CAFETERIA

Tips:

- ♥ Take a look at the whole cafeteria line before going through. That way, you can have your menu planned out.
- ♥ Cafeterias often add margarine to cooked vegetables, though you can ask that all the juices be strained from your portion.

♥ Call ahead to see if your cafeteria carries any fat-free condiments--if not, bring your own. Also ask how some of your favorite foods are prepared.

♥ There are usually several fruit salads that have no fat added.

♥ If you can't resist the temptation of seeing all the high-fat foods, you should stay away from cafeterias!

Suggested Menus:

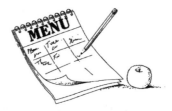

- Strawberry and banana salad
- Steamed broccoli
- New potatoes
- Carrot coins
- Pinto beans
- Cornbread

- Fruited jello
- Frozen fruit salad
- Spinach
- Black-eyed peas
- Okra and tomatoes

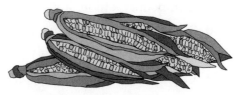

- Three bean salad
- Spaghetti with marinara Sauce
- Steamed zuchinni and yellow squash
- Fresh fruit salad

PIZZA

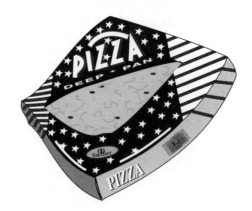

Tips:

♥ Order your pizza without cheese--for most people the crust is the best part anyway!

♥ Ask that they use no additional oil on the top or bottom.

♥ Top your pizza with all the veggies and sauce you desire!

♥ If you order your pizza delivered or get it "take out," you can add a bit of fat-free mozzarella or parmesan cheese to it when you get home.

Suggested Toppings:

🍎 Bell pepper, onion, mushroom

🍎 Tomato or extra tomato sauce

🍎 Olive (if put on sparingly)

🍎 Capers (you can add this at home)

🍎 Pineapple

🍎 Any other vegetables

ALL YOU CAN EAT BUFFETS

Someone is cashing in on American's desire to get their money's worth when it comes to the dinner bill. If you have "eyes that are bigger than your stomach" at these places, you might want to choose a different sort of restaurant in which to dine. I was pleasantly surprised to find that Country Buffet had two fat-free salad dressings to choose from and fat-free frozen yogurt for dessert. Good Choices:

- ❤ Carrots
- ❤ Baked beans
- ❤ Corn
- ❤ Fruit salad

- ❤ Mashed potatoes
- ❤ Green beans
- ❤ Salad bar (see page 133)
- ❤ Rolls

STEAK HOUSES

Most steak houses offer salads or a salad bar, baked potato, rice and some type of fresh vegetables. Some offer a large salad bar extravaganza, which contains a lot more than just salad. A good lowfat meal can be had at a steak restaurant, especially one with a "food bar." However, first you must be able to pass up the steaks and all the fried foods available on the "food bar." If you can't, it's safer to stick with restaurants with fewer temptations.

BEST BETS--CHAIN RESTAURANTS

All the dinner menus listed below contain 12 grams of fat or less. Dinner menus were chosen, assuming that most people eat a larger dinner.

♥ *Applebee's*
  - ♦ Steamed Vegetable and Salad plate (hold the cheese & bacon) bring your own dressing

♥ *Bennigan's*
  - ♦ Steamed vegetable platter
  - ♦ Baked potato
  - ♦ Spinach side salad (hold the bacon & eggs)
  - ♦ Bread (hold the butter)

♥ *Chili's*

Chili's has a number of offerings for the heart-conscious eater; fat-free dressings, a lowfat vegetarian entree, some lowfat side dishes and even fat-free frozen yogurt. You can have a tasty meal here
  - ♦ Side salad with no fat Honey Mustard Dressing
  - ♦ Guiltless Veggie Pasta
  - ♦ Southwest Sling Smoothie (Nonfat vanilla yogurt, pineapple juice, orange juice and strawberries)

♥ *Big Boy Restaurant and Bake Shop*
  - ♦ Vegetable Stir fry with rice
  - ♦ Roll
  - ♦ Fat-Free Frozen Yogurt

♥ *California Pizza Kitchen*
  - ♦ Grilled Eggplant, Thai or Vegetarian Pizza (all cheese-less
  - ♦ Field Greens Salad (bring own dressing)

♥ *Denny's*
  - ♦ Garden salad (bring own dressing)
  - ♦ Carrots and green beans
  - ♦ Bowl split pea soup
  - ♦ Corn and peas
  - ♦ Plain baked potato
  - ♦ Toasted Bagel

♥ *Olive Garden*

- 🍎 Garden salad (bring own dressing or use vinegar)
- 🍎 Minestrone soup
- 🍎 Spaghetti with marinara Sauce

♥ *Red Lobster*

- 🍎 Rice pilaf or baked potato
- 🍎 Fresh vegetables (hold butter sauce)
- 🍎 Dinner salad with lite Italian dressing
- 🍎 Sherbet

♥ *TGI Friday's*

On a recent "research trip" to Friday's, I was impressed with their offerings, including 4 vegetarian selections and 2 tasty fat-free dressings. For dessert, try a Fling--a fruit drink.

- 🍎 Garden Burger
- 🍎 Fresh Vegetable Baguette (hold the swiss cheese
- 🍎 House salad (hold the garlic bread) with fat-free Italian herb dressing

♥ *Red Robin*

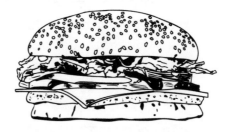

- 🍎 Meatless burger
- 🍎 Side salad with fat-free dressing instead of french fries
- 🍎 Steamer basket; vegetables and pasta with fat-free dressing

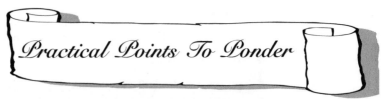

Practical Points To Ponder

EATING RIGHT WHILE TRAVELING

- ♥ When flying, call the airline at least 24 hours in advance to order a lowfat vegetarian meal.

- ♥ Bring snacks such as pretzels, fresh fruit, and granola bars to fill in--airline food is getting mighty skimpy!

- ♥ Before making your hotel reservation, find out if healthy food choices are available at their restaurants. It's also wise to find a hotel that has a pool or fitness room.

- ♥ Reserve a hotel room with a refrigerator and / or cooking facilities. Having a refrigerator will allow you to have a fat-free breakfast in your room and healthy snacks for between meals.

- ♥ Try to go to a grocery store upon arrival to buy healthy foods. If staying with friends or relatives, this will ease the burden of them providing the foods you need or you eating foods you shouldn't out of guilt.

- ♥ Dine at the chain restaurants mentioned above that you know will have healthy food choices.

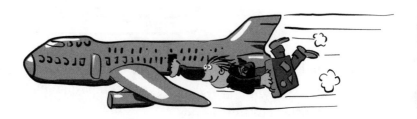

CHAPTER 7

WOMEN AND HEART DISEASE--THE WEAKER SEX?

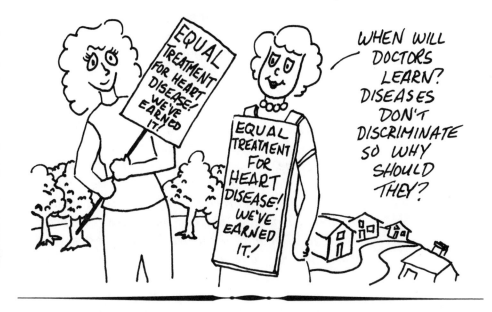

"All's fair in love and war."

HEART DISEASE AND STROKE are the leading causes of death among American women. Last year, over 485,000 women died from these preventable illnesses. I'd like to tell you about one of these women.

> *My patient, Mrs. M, had just gone through the menopause. I was out of town when she rushed to the Emergency Department, complaining of weakness and difficulty breathing. An evaluation, including a complete pelvic exam showed anemia from vaginal bleeding. She was admitted to the Women's Pavilion of the hospital.*

The next morning, I visited Mrs. M. "I feel lousy, like an elephant is sitting on my chest!" And she looked lousy--pale, sweating, gasping for air, she appeared very sick. A quick look through her chart showed only the anemia, now corrected with blood transfusions. No ECG had been performed to check the heart. No chest X-ray to check the lungs. No oxygen given for the breathing. Her heart wasn't even being monitored!

The "stat" ECG came as a shock. It clearly showed evidence of a major heart attack! By good fortune alone, she was stabilized in the coronary care unit with medical therapy. Although fluid filled her lungs, powerful water pills soon made her lose 10 pounds. Oxygen and digoxin helped boost the strength of the heart. However, extensive heart damage had been done.

The next day, after her heart catheterization showed blockages in all three main heart arteries and not amenable to bypass surgery, she asked me the inevitable question. "Why did this happen to me? I lost my husband last year. I'm getting ready to retire. I deserve a better fate!"

Of course, she was right. Feeling sick with anguish, I mulled over an answer. Mentally I reviewed her risk factors: former heavy smoker, overweight, lack of exercise, and the stress of losing her spouse. Although I didn't have an adequate answer, I stressed the future and hope for a recovery.

Several weeks later Mrs. M made an office visit. She was feeling improved after cardiac rehabilitation, but still wasn't her old self. "My daughter invited me to see <u>Phantom of the Opera</u>. I very much want to go!" I knew the theatre steps were many and steep. However, after she passed her treadmill exercise test, I agreed she could go.

I waited somewhat apprehensively for a call that weekend, but none came. Later in the week, she did call to say she had the best time ever, and no troubles at all! We were both very relieved.

It was a month later that the next call came. Mrs. M was found in her car, dead, by the side of the road. The coroner determined she had suffered a second heart attack, but was in enough control to get off the busy street and stop the car, saving other lives in the process.

Mrs. M taught me many lessons about women and heart disease, lessons I want to share with you now.

IS THERE SEX BIAS IN THE TREATMENT OF HEART DISEASE?

Certainly, there is no bias in Mother Nature. Slightly more women than men have heart disease, and more women than men die yearly from heart disease and stroke (485,000 a year).

For decades, medical research was an "old boy's club," run by men on male subjects only. The standard medical viewpoint was that heart disease was more prevalent in men. The proof? All the studies said so. When women were finally admitted into the research studies, the true extent of heart disease in women was discovered. Still the myths persisted.

More recently, research has shown further, shocking disparities between the sexes. When men and women with chest pain were evaluated in emergency departments, twice as many men were admitted and received further evaluation and therapy. (Reference 30)

Even after sophisticated heart testing in men and women which was all positive for heart disease, men received further and more aggressive intervention than women. (Reference 31)

A higher proportion of first heart attacks are fatal in women, 8% more than in men. Additionally, women are several times more likely than men to die after bypass surgery.

It seems that men and women are evaluated and treated differently, even today. Controversy persists as to why, but there is general agreement that there is a bias.

RISK FACTORS

The factors causing heart disease are well known. Women share many of the same risk factors as men:

♥ Smoking

- ♥ High blood pressure
- ♥ High cholesterol
- ♥ Lack of exercise
- ♥ Stress
- ♥ Obesity

However, there are several persisting differences in women:

- ♥ More diabetes
- ♥ Higher incidence of congestive heart failure
- ♥ Dramatic increase in risk after the menopause
- ♥ More "atypical angina", less typical activity related chest pain
- ♥ For those having a heart attack, a much worse prognosis, based on diffuse and severe coronary artery disease
- ♥ Greater risk of death after bypass surgery

THE MENOPAUSE

No serious discussion of women's issues would be adequate without including the menopause. As the aging of America continues, women live nearly half their lives after going through the "change of life." This causes many effects, some of which are related to the absence of female hormones. The largest effect: increased cardiovascular disease and death.

Estrogen is one of the two principal female hormones, the other being progesterone. Estrogen is known to protect women from increased rates of heart disease after the menopause. In the huge **Nurses Health Study**, postmenopausal estrogen decreased the risk of heart disease by half. The good effects were evident even after adjustments were made for the other standard risk factors. (Reference 32)

Much of this protection is mediated through higher levels of HDL, the "good cholesterol" (Reference 33), as well as through other mechanisms. Users of estrogen after the menopause have lower rates of death (35%) from all causes than nonusers.

THE FEAR FACTOR

Other issues are raised when studying the estrogen replacement question. One that receives very little recognition or discussion is what I term "the fear factor." This is the notion that anything which could influence contracting "THE BIG C" (cancer) is a fate worse than death. Many women, motivated by this fear, disregard or refuse out of hand therapy which could improve their health.

We already know that heart disease is the biggest killer of women. One in seven women 45 to 64 years old has some form of coronary heart disease. Over 485,000 women die a year. Compare that to **all forms** of cancer deaths in women, at 233,000. Estrogen reduces the risk of heart disease by half. The fear factor is an important consideration in the health and well-being of women. Let's examine the facts of estrogen replacement after the menopause. And let's do away with the myths.

OSTEOPOROSIS

Hip fractures occur at a rate of 280,000 a year. Deaths from this disease approach 30,000 yearly.

Prevention includes improved diet, weight-bearing exercise, and smoking cessation. Additionally, estrogen therapy is very effective in preserving the strength of the bones after the menopause. The risk of hip fracture can be reduced by up to 60% (Reference 34).

PREVENTING OSTEOPOROSIS: CALCIUM

How much do we need, how can we get it into our bones, and what are the best sources of the mineral?

National Institute of Health panel published guidelines on optimal levels of calcium; which vary with age and sex--see table 9.

Group	Daily Calcium Intake mg.
Men:	
25-65 years	1000
Over 65 years	1500
Women:	
25-50 years	1000
Over 50 years; Post-menopause:	
Taking estrogen	1000
Not on estrogen	1500
Over 65 years	1500

Table 9. Optimal Calcium Intake (Reference 35)

So, if we all need calcium, what is the best way to absorb it without side effects? Vitamin D is necessary, and is available through sunlight, fortified foods, and supplements.

From 400 IU will do the trick. For food sources of calcium, which are absorbed very efficiently, see table 10.

SOURCES OF CALCIUM

Food item	Calcium in mg.
Firm tofu (If made with calcium), raw, 1 cup:	517
Tums	500
Yogurt, fat-free plain, 1 cup	452
Yogurt, fat-free vanilla, 1 cup	400
Wonder enriched bread, 1 slice	290
Tropicana orange juice plus calcium, 1 cup	333
Skim milk, 1 cup	302
Minute Maid enriched orange juice, 1 cup	293
Amaranth (grain), 1 cup	276
Collards, frozen, cooked: 1 cup	358
Figs, 1/2 cup	143
Baked beans, 1 cup	139
Turnip greens, frozen, cooked, 1 cup	250
Sherbet, 1 cup	103
Kale, 1 cup	180
Soybeans, 1 cup	176
Bok choy, 1/2 cup	79

Table 10. Calcium sources

After the menopause, there is one very important thing you can do to "build strong bones twelve ways." Consider taking estrogen. At the menopause, a woman's body begins to leach calcium from old bone at a fast pace. This affects the wrist and spine the most. And age itself has the effect of slowing the pace of new bone growth. This affects the hips. Estrogen replacement has a major effect on retarding this bone loss.

Don't forget the beneficial effects of exercise on building strong bones. Weight-bearing exercise can build and preserve bone mass, thus preventing osteoporosis. In conjunction with estrogen and calcium, this is the most effective prevention program for osteoporosis.

ENDOMETRIAL CANCER

Estrogen can cause cancer of the endometrium (lining of the womb) when used alone. It causes about 5,900 deaths a year (Reference 36). If found early, it can be cured by removing the uterus (hysterectomy). Let's look at the numbers:

Study group	Cancer per 100,000 per year
Estrogen only users	390
No hormones	245
Estrogen + Progesterone	49
All groups combined	113

Table 11. Number of Endometrial Cancers

Using the combination of hormones dramatically **decreases the risk of cancer of the endometrium**. It also gives the added benefit of heart disease protection to a very susceptible population of women (Reference 37). If you have had a hysterectomy (Removal of the uterus), you need only take estrogen.

BREAST CANCER

No other cancer causes the fear factor in women like breast cancer. It is so common that most women have a friend or relative stricken with it. After the age of 50 or so, corresponding to menopause, the incidence rises dramatically. If all cases are included, even in 80 to 90 year old women dying of other causes, about 1 in 12 women will develop breast cancer. It is estimated that 145,000 new cases are found each year, and it causes 46,000 death a year. Most breast cancers occur at advanced age.

Breast cancer is the second most common cancer in women, after cancer of the lung. It is associated with a high-fat diet. There is no convincing evidence that breast cancer is caused by post-menopausal estrogen replacement (Reference 38). There is controversy about pre-menopausal effects of estrogen on the development of breast cancer. For those **with** breast cancer, estrogen can stimulate its growth.

There is evidence that a combination of estrogen and progesterone may decrease the incidence of breast cancer, similar to the situation with the endometrium (Reference 37).

Realizing that risks for breast cancer vary, it seems prudent to sustain a lowfat meal plan to prevent this common disease. If you have very close family history (mother or sister with breast cancer) you can be tested for the breast cancer gene. You can discuss other ways to sustain your health, such as post-menopausal estrogen replacement, with your personal physician.

ESTROGEN REPLACEMENT THERAPY--WHAT TO DO?

On balance, the numbers clearly indicate tremendous benefit with estrogen and progesterone use. Numbers, however, clearly don't address "the fear factor." On this deeply personal level, several issues are important.

❤ During the prime of your life, from menopause to age 80, heart disease and associated deaths greatly outnumber breast cancer.

❤ The factors causing heart disease are well known, and many can be modified.

❤ The factors causing breast cancer are less well known although fat in the diet can also be modified.

❤ Can we, as a society, allow women, because of misinformation, to continue to die with heart disease rather than face the fear factor of breast cancer?

❤ Does the issue of osteoporosis (thin, fragile bones) influence your thinking? Estrogen and a lowfat, high calcium diet have been proven to prevent this disease of women.

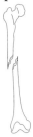

❤ If you don't take estrogen, a lowfat diet can empower you to help prevent both heart disease and cancer.

These issues are not easy. Please consult your personal physician for a detailed examination and discussion before deciding on the hormone replacement issue.

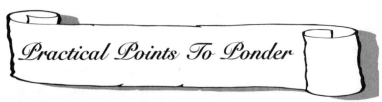

Practical Points To Ponder

TAKE CHARGE OF YOUR HEALTH CARE

♥ Reduce your risk factors for heart disease:
  ◆ Stop smoking
  ◆ Eat right, cut out the fat
  ◆ Exercise regularly

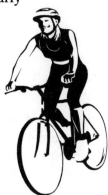

  ◆ Check your blood pressure and cholesterol
♥ If you have signs or symptoms of heart disease, such as chest pain, shortness of breath, fatigue, night sweats, or others, see your doctor immediately!
♥ After your examination, don't accept "it's all in your head" as an adequate explanation. Demand a full and careful inquiry into the cause of your symptoms. If your doctor balks, or doesn't treat disease if found, find another doctor!
♥ You **can** prevent and reverse heart disease! Make up your mind, and MAKE THE CHANGE!

CHAPTER 8	# *SO WHAT'S STOPPING YOU?*

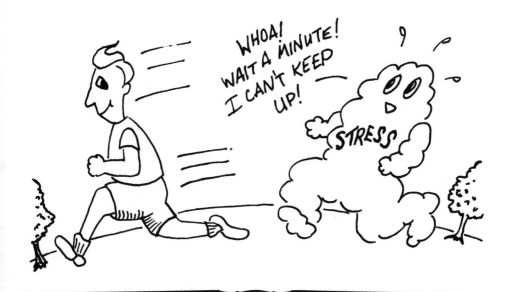

"If you can't stand the heat, get out of the kitchen."

Harry S. Truman

STRESS, AND HOW TO BEAT IT!

A cardiac patient of mine, a rather young man to have a heart attack, decided to go through the Preventive Health Institute program after his recuperation. He did well, felt better, lost weight, and lowered his cholesterol and blood pressure. However, he kept complaining about the stress of his job. "It's killing me" Joe said with a smile. "I can't keep up with the demands."

Six months later I saw Joe in the office. His face was bloated. The blood pressure was sky high, as was his cholesterol. He had gained weight. I asked him what happened.

"It's the job. It's killing me! I can't take the stress. I've even considered retiring, but I feel the others would think less of me as a person. Like I was a quitter."

We discussed finances, pressure, health, and a host of other things. The issue was unresolved when he left. His biggest issue seemed to be the sense of failure he felt with quitting his job. As if he had to continue at all costs, no matter what the personal price.

We had spoken of priorities. Joe did take the time to sit with his wife and make a list. It was emotional at times. Finally, they agreed on goals for the next several years.

One month later, Joe kept his scheduled appointment. As I walked in, he was smiling! "I'm retiring! And even though I have 6 months left, I feel like a weight has been lifted from my shoulders. I feel like a new man." He certainly was acting like a new man. He had beaten stress!

The very fortunate part of Joe's story is that, from then on, he found positive health changes much easier to accomplish. And I'm pleased to report, Joe is a happy and healthy man today.

THIRTY-FIVE WAYS TO LEAVE YOUR STRESS

(to the tune of "Fifty Ways To Leave Your Lover" by Paul Simon)

1. Take a walk in the rain.
2. Take a walk in the rain, holding hands.
3. Tried riding a bike, lately? You never forget how.
4. Hike up your favorite hill.
5. Swim your troubles away.

6. Have sex often.
7. Join a group, any group.
8. Turn off the TV and find time to join a group.
9. Enjoy a good belly laugh.
10. Offer to help someone else more in need than you are.

11. Think positive.
12. Take control of your work stresses.
13. Be realistic. How bad is the worst thing you fear?
14. Live in the present. No one is good at seeing the future.
15. Bend a little, change a little. Perhaps a yoga class?

16. Stretch your neck and shoulders.
17. Learn a relaxation technique.
18. Listen to music you enjoy.
19. Practice deep breathing.

20. Take a break, even for five minutes.

21. Read a good book.
22. "Don't sweat the small stuff" because...
23. "Everything is the small stuff."
24. Play Santa Claus this year.
25. Take a lunch break each day at work.

26. Learn to "problem solve"
27. Change a behavior that causes more worry than it helps.
28. Speak up. Others don't know if you are worried.
29. Pick up a hobby or sport that requires concentration.
30. Lower your shoulders once an hour to relax.

31. Explore your spiritual side.
32. Visit the church of your upbringing.
33. Invest 5 minutes a day daydreaming.
34. Take up a new sport.
35. Dance.

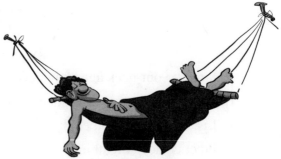

STRESS REDUCTION USUALLY COMES DOWN TO

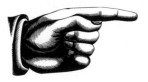

- ♥ Exercise
- ♥ Getting connected with others
- ♥ Positive mental attitude
- ♥ Self control, mind over matter

Your heart can't take the stress. Why?

I have a short story about my father. He was a smoker. A veteran of World War II, he worked for years at IBM. When it came time for me to graduate from Georgetown University, he had just finished a Master's degree from New York University. Because, I think, of the stress of job, school, and the added financial pressure of a son headed to medical school, his heart attack came quickly and unexpectedly. The morning of graduation, he couldn't finish breakfast. The attack was fatal. He was 53. I believe stress did him in.

Some people are termed "hot reactors." They pay a high price for stress because their blood pressure rises to high levels, **without their awareness**. Over time, the heart suffers greatly.

The good news: this bodily reaction can be unlearned. And this is fortuitous, because stress may be the single most important factor in recurring heart problems. Let me tell you what we see at the Preventive Health Institute. And how to change it!

- A recent study (Reference 39) proved that mental stress constricted the coronary arteries as much or more than smoking and cocaine use!

- Another study (Reference 40) showed that men with high anxiety are six times more likely than calmer men to have sudden cardiac death.

- Depression in heart patients is a better predictor of future heart events than severity of heart damage, high cholesterol, and smoking (Reference 41).

THE SINGLE MOST IMPORTANT PROBLEM WE CHANGE AT THE PREVENTIVE HEALTH INSTITUTE IS NOT HEART DISEASE. IT'S THE STRESS THAT LED TO THE HEART DISEASE. IT'S THE STRESS THAT BLOCKS THE CHANGES NECESSARY TO GET HEALTHY.

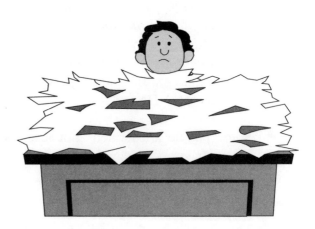

Take the following "Life Event Test" and rate your stress level. This may be the most important heart-related test you take! (Note: good stress and bad stress both affect you.)

LIFE EVENT TEST

LIFE EVENT	POINTS	TOTAL
Death of a spouse	100	____
Divorce	73	____
Marital separation	65	____
Jail term	63	____
Death of a close family member	63	____
Personal injury or illness	53	____
Marriage	50	____
Fired at work	47	____
Marital reconciliation	45	____
Retirement	45	____
Change in a family member's health	44	____
Pregnancy	40	____
Sex difficulties	39	____
Addition to family	39	____
Business readjustment	39	____
Change in financial state	38	____
Death of a close friend	37	____
Change to a different line of work	36	____
Change in number of marital arguments	35	____
Loan for a major purchase	31	____
Foreclosure	30	____
Kids leaving home	29	____
Trouble with in-laws	29	____
Outstanding personal achievement	28	____
Finishing school	26	____
Change in living conditions	25	____
Trouble with boss	23	____
Change in work hours	20	____
Change in residence	20	____
Change in schools	20	____

TOTAL SCORE ____

Your score:

- ♥ 300 or greater: 80% chance of illness in the near future
- ♥ 150 to 299: 50% chance of illness
- ♥ less than 150: about 30% chance of illness

(Reprinted with permission from *Journal of Psychosomatic Research*, vol.11, pages 213-218, 1967, "The Social Readjustment Rating Scale", Elsevier Science Ltd., Pergamon Imprint, Oxford, England)

ANGER

Anger is a common manifestation of depression, stress or anxiety. We all know people who are "always angry." I'd like to tell you about Gene. Gene was a "pain in the butt." Nothing was ever good enough. Nary a kind word passed his lips. The group was fed up!

Don't ask me why, but at one group session, Gene raised his hand. "You people just don't understand. I saw it all in Vietnam! My buddies on the ground blown away. Some wounded so badly life wasn't worth living. Every time I hear the sound of a helicopter or plane, I duck and break out in a cold sweat. They won't get a chance to burn me ever again! I know, it makes me a terrible grouch, but I don't know any other way."

Did this outburst cure Gene's anger? Not a chance. However, after the group, another fellow befriended Gene. He, too, was a Vietnam War veteran, but had a slightly different perspective on life. They struck up a conversation, and quite a friendship.

The group noticed some subtle changes in Gene. The edges were still there, but perhaps not so sharp. Gene's explanation, which he shared with me months later--"I finally felt understood." He seemed less angry. He also seemed much more connected with people.

STEPS FOR CONTROLLING ANGER

- ♥ Stop, "I'm getting angry."
- ♥ Think about what will happen if you lose control.
  "If I lose control..."
- ♥ Ask yourself why you're really angry.
  "The real reason I'm angry is..."
- ♥ Reduce anger. "I need to cool down, I'm going to..."
- ♥ Reward yourself. "I did a good job. I'm going to..."

EXPRESSING ANGER

- ♥ Tell the person how you feel. "I'm..."
- ♥ Identify the specific event that made you feel that way.
  "I'm... because..."
- ♥ Explain why you feel that way. "When you... I feel..."

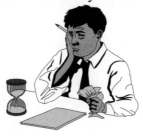

CONTROLLING YOUR INNER SELF

Try the following relaxation techniques daily. The more you practice, the better it works. And, it will be ready for you in times of increased stress.

Start under optimal conditions--a quiet comfortable room, where you will not be disturbed. As you improve your concentration, practice in other more public places. Before too long, you'll be able to practice self-control anywhere!

RELAXATION PRACTICE TECHNIQUES

♥ **Two-minute body stress scanning** can be extended when you have the time. People often do this when they must wait; while watching TV, during traffic, or while in a line.

♦ Interrupt your thoughts, stop thinking about your surroundings and switch your thoughts to your breathing. Using the diaphragm, take two deep breaths and exhale **slowly**.

♦ Scan yourself for tense or uncomfortable spots: forehead? jaw? shoulders? Attempt to loosen this area up a little. Allow your muscles to feel as heavy and warm as they can in this amount of time.

♦ Warm your hands momentarily.

♦ Do two quick yoga exercises:

Rotate your head around in a circular motion once or twice.

Roll your shoulders forward and backward a couple of times.

♦ Recall a pleasant thought, image, memory, or feeling just for a few seconds.

♦ Take another **deep breath** from the diaphragm and return to your activities.

♥ **The Quieting Response** is designed to last 10 seconds, but can be extended when you wish. This is a good exercise to use in the midst of chaos, panic, hectic circumstances, or times when you feel you can only spare less than a minute.

   ♦ Quickly determine what it is about this situation, here and now, that is annoying. (For example, the phone might be ringing frequently, there may be excessive noise, etc.)

   ♦ **Smile** (outwardly or inwardly) and say to yourself, "leave my body out of this." This can either be aloud or to yourself.

   ♦ Take two easy deep breaths. As you inhale count from 1 to 4, and as you exhale count from 1 to 4.

   ♦ As you exhale the second breath, let your jaw go limp, and quickly spread some of this relaxed, loose feeling to other tense muscle groups.

   ♦ Resume your activities.

♥ **A Short Meditation**

   ♦ First scan your body, see what your muscles feel like, attempt to relax and loosen up, allow yourself to feel body sensations. Stay with this body scanning for a couple of minutes. Allow the muscles to feel as heavy and warm as possible. Focus on warmth in your arms and hands.

   ♦ Focus now on your thoughts. What are you thinking of? What kinds of thoughts have you had today, and which ones "come to mind" now? Are these upsetting thoughts or comforting ones? Dwell on the comforting or pleasant thoughts--place a greater emphasis on these thoughts.

♦ Focus now on your emotions or feelings. What do you feel? Content? Angry? Annoyed? Sad? Excited? Peaceful? Allow yourself to feel.

♦ Take 3 deep breaths (easy and slow) and return to your activities.

Practice these techniques daily!

GET ON THE STICK!

MOTIVATION

Motivation is the inner drive that compels you to behave in a certain way. When you have motivation, you have (the tools for) it all!

The easiest patients I care for are the ones with a large, built-in reserve of motivation. They are high-performance athletes even though they may not be in the Olympics or even participate in an organized sport. Injury or illness is seen by them as a temporary obstacle or barrier to their continued athletic performance. For instance:

Three months of rehab? "I bet I can do it in two!"

This is a very complicated disease? "Doctor, you tell me exactly what I need to do to get better, and I'll do it. I'm not your usual patient. I want to get well!"

What we know about motivation

- ♥ Knowledge alone is not enough to motivate a long term change in your behavior.

- ♥ Aversion technique (can be somewhat helpful) is training the mind and body to be repelled by a negative addiction. i.e. smoking.

- ♥ Incentive technique (which works best at changing long term behaviors) is rewarding with something pleasurable after accomplishing positive behavior.

- ♥ Different types of motivation work for different people.

SEVEN SURE-FIRE WAYS TO IMPROVE MOTIVATION!

...Identify your CORE GOALS or DESIRES, the things or actions or wants that only you know are most important to you.

Core desires are genuine, clearly defined **wants** that cause you to be willing to put forth the effort necessary to make your desire become a reality. This even means overcoming seemingly insurmountable obstacles.

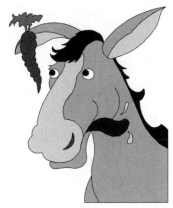

CORE DESIRES, once defined by you, can be used to activate the inherent motivation to achieve CORE DESIRE that **YOU** get from "within." Your "coach" or physician can help you develop your core desires, but only **YOU** can have them.

♥ DISCOVER YOUR OWN CORE DESIRE

Example: Being fit, if a priority, may bring you

...Physical attractiveness

...Love and laughter of friends

...Enhanced stamina

But how do you realize what these desires are? It starts with being honest with yourself. If you can get through the layers of excuses and explanations and negative thoughts many of us have, you are on your way to being truly honest with yourself.

Then what? It will take an honest effort and a little time to "brainstorm" a short list of the **really important things**. We suggest sitting down with a spouse, friend, clergyman or counselor to generate a short list. Give yourself several hours, and remember, it's not written in stone. Give yourself permission to go back and revise before settling on your true goals.

♥ BRING YOUR CORE DESIRE TO THE SURFACE WITH DAILY ACKNOWLEDGEMENT

Unfortunately, if you don't think about it often, it may slip from your grasp. With the hustle and bustle of daily life, we have plenty of thoughts crowding into our daily consciousness. Some suggestions for keeping the most important "up front":

...Post a message to yourself where you will see and read it daily

...Take a photograph of what you want the "new you" to look like and display it prominently. Alternatively, get a photograph of someone you respect or want to emulate and look at it often.

...Use the bathroom mirror to look yourself straight in the eye, and affirm your new goals.

♥ ACTIVELY REPLACE OLD BELIEFS ABOUT CORE DESIRE WITH NEW POSITIVE ONES

For instance, replace "I've never been very physical" with "Exercise boosts my energy level!" Then go about restructuring your beliefs. Instead of "I'd rather die than walk in the rain," think about "Singing in the Rain" and how incredibly romantic it might be, with the right company.

Another example we hear frequently at the Preventive Health Institute revolves around food. "I could never live without meat" frequently becomes, "most of the time, I feel better when I eat healthy food. I still like to splurge on the big holidays, however."

♥ IDENTIFY THE OUTCOMES OF CORE DESIRES

This step can help to further define behaviors that can get you where you want to go. For example, if a global desire is better health, break it down into results: lower blood pressure, improved sleep patterns, increased energy, stress release, enhanced self esteem.

Try the traditional "I want to win the lottery." Then take it one step further. If indeed you had "lots" of money, what exactly would you do?

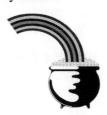

Make The Change For A Healthy Heart   **175**

♥ WHEN THE IMPULSE TO DROP OUT IS OVER-WHELMING, SIMPLY DROP DOWN INSTEAD

Sticking to anything new is NOT easy over the long haul. There is a built in pessimism about trying again, perhaps a sense of failure. Realize your humanity! Life has its ebbs and flows... iron clad consistency is not for every-one. For example, it takes an average of three tries to stop smoking. We all know of someone who was successful!

Start again, by repeating the previous steps. Make sure your goals are realistic. After all, if you need hamburgers once a week rather than once a month, you are still a lot better off than twice a day! And you still have the option of reevaluating and changing again in the future. As we say at the Preventive Health Institute, "it's very hard to see the future."

♥ BECOME AN EXCUSE BUSTER BY NOT MEETING THE EXCUSE HEAD ON, BUT BY SIDE STEPPING IT

For example, if you have started to believe "I hate driv-ing to the gym"--then tell yourself "Nobody said I had to." Consider buying exercise equipment for home use. Try to reprogram yourself! Think differently!

Avoid the negative by creating a positive thought or situ-ation instead. DON'T let a lapse become a permanent relapse!

♥ DIFFERENT DRIVES FOR DIFFERENT LIVES, or different strokes for different folks!

Motivation is not necessarily born of logic, knowledge, or experience. It is locked within you, and you carry the combination.

Investigating what motivates you allows you to look at what triggers your behavior.

WHY DO WE FAIL TO ACHIEVE GOALS?????

- ♥ Most people start with impossible or unrealistic goals - "I want to win the lottery." This is often seen in the sports world, where a young athlete may voice a desire to be in the Olympics. A trained coach, however, constantly tries to break success down into its components, i.e. "Why don't you spend time **practicing** hitting the curve ball this week?"

- ♥ Striving to reach someone else's goal: spouses, parents.

- ♥ If the goal isn't really important to you, isn't your "core desire," it's easy to sabotage the goal.

- ♥ Little or no desire to achieve goal. If it's easier to stay where you are, you will!

- ♥ Lack of Self-Awareness. So many of us don't know what we want out of life. It's easier to reach a place if you know where you're headed.

- ♥ Not measuring goals... What, how much, when. How will you gauge if you're improving. Batting average going up? Cholesterol dropping? Energy better? A's on the report card?

- ♥ Lack of Visualization. If you don't know what the new, slim, trim, self-confident you will be like, you may be too afraid to make the change. Change often is scary.

- ♥ Lack of Affirmation. "I am better or healthier, or thinner, today than I was yesterday" Say the words, repeat them, over and over.

- ♥ No Reward system. "I lost those pounds, I deserve the new clothes." If change isn't going to translate into something tangible in your life, why do it?

STAGES OF CHANGE

Everyone goes through these stages, like a spiral, from one to the other, as the circumstances of our lives change. Try to pick out, for several health related behaviors, what stage you are in presently.

Precontemplation: Not intending to change a behavior in the foreseeable future. You do not yet care enough about this behavior to consider change.

Contemplation: Intending to change a behavior in the foreseeable future (next 6 months, but not the immediate future. Good, at least you're thinking about it!

Preparation: Planning to change a behavior in the near future (next 30 days) and taking some steps toward change. Plan to do it during a low stress time.

Action: You have recently changed the behavior, or have tried and failed, but not given up. For example, quitting smoking usually takes two or three tries. Keep at it!

Maintenance: Changed the behavior for greater than six months. You succeed, one day at a time.

After Procheska, *"The Transtheoretical Model"* (Reference 42)

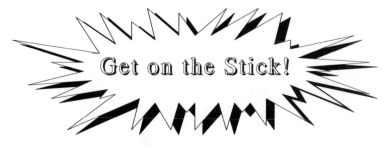

Get on the Stick!

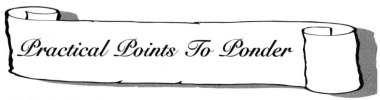

MOTIVATION

- ♥ Discover your core desire or goal.
- ♥ Acknowledge it daily.
- ♥ Think positive. The power of positive thinking is one of those things that must be first believed, then you will see it!
- ♥ Where do you want to be for the rest of your life?
- ♥ Don't drop out, drop down.
- ♥ Side step excuses.
- ♥ Different strokes for different folks. What motivates you?

CHEATING

Here's a little story about food!

> *One of our participants at the Preventive Health Institute, let's call him Dan, was having a rough time. He had suffered two cardiac arrests and several heart attacks. After a new, experimental surgery, he had stabilized. He still struggled with his weight and cholesterol.*

> *Dan was having a hard time with the concept of meat as a high-fat food. "I just love the smell of a*

barbecue. I rinse the hamburger, and dry it on paper towels. Then I partially cook it in a frying pan, and throw away the liquid fat. Finally, I broil it. Anything wrong with that?"

We spent several sessions in the group talking with Dan. People were very interested to know why he spent so much time and effort for one little burger.

It was several weeks later, when we were enjoying a dinner of "non-meat" vegetarian burgers, buns, and all the toppings, that we found out. "This is great! Just what I enjoy. The smell, summertime, good conversation with friends. And these are a lot easier to make!" He later admitted he just was being stubborn, not wanting to admit the seriousness of his heart problems, and the burgers made him feel independent from his disease. Yes, once a month, Dan still needs a veggie burger on the grill. He has been able to make many, daily, healthy changes without his independence feeling threatened!

- ♥ Who are you cheating?
  - ♦ Yourself, always. As you know, a treat or a feast on a special occasion "feels" different from cheating. It's that feeling you should attend to.
  - ♦ Are you sometimes mad at the boss, and instead of telling the boss, you eat?
  - ♦ Have there been stressful family interactions? A family member can be hard to confront. Do you take it out on food instead?

- ♥ Why are you cheating?
    - ◆ Angry at someone? Stressed?
    - ◆ No other reward system?
    - ◆ Feeling self-destructive? or Depressed?
    - ◆ Scorned or spurned?
    - ◆ Lonely?
    - ◆ Or, like Dan, having trouble accepting the reality of your present situation?
- ♥ The key to the puzzle: why do you eat, why do you make harmful choices. Eating is much more symbolic than filling the belly and getting energy from food. Just look at our major holidays! The big event usually revolves around eating, and in the USA, overeating!
- ♥ You can eat more food on a lowfat meal plan.
- ♥ You can help your emotional state by dealing with it, rather than smothering it with food!

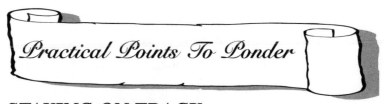

Practical Points To Ponder

STAYING ON TRACK

- ♥ If you have heart disease and "cheat" more than once a month, you may need to examine stress, emotions, purpose in life.
- ♥ If you are trying to be supportive to someone following the program, but "cheat" more than once a week, you may be undermining your loved one. This is termed "enabling" behavior.

♥ Other ways to avoid cheating

Plan ahead. If you have plenty of lowfat, healthy food available, burgers and pizza will be less tempting.

Drink lots of water.

Exercise daily.

Have plenty of snacks available. Use them.

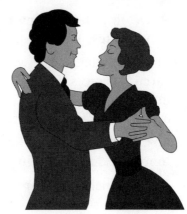

♥ Healthy snacks to keep you from feeling like "cheating":

Fat-free cookies

Fruit: raisins, apples, bananas, oranges

Popcorn: a bushel full!

Fat-free pretzels: Rold Gold, Mr. Phipps

Angel food cake

Fat-free frozen yogurt

Vegetables: carrots, celery, cherry tomatoes

lowfat bread and honey or jam, or bagels

Rice cakes: Quaker Oats

We are all human and make mistakes. Let's try to minimize them. If we don't learn from our mistakes, we will be doomed to repeat them forever!

CHAPTER 9

MOVE YOUR BODY

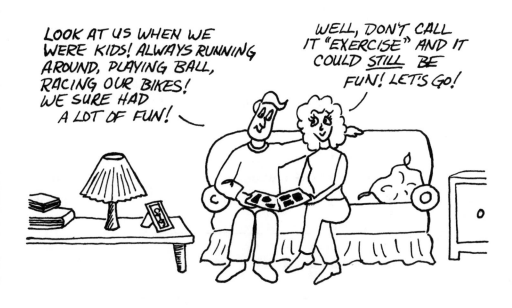

"If you don't move it, you lose it!"

Some people with heart disease fear that exercise might hurt them. As we will show, exercise will help your heart and attitude.

RATE YOUR FITNESS LEVEL

What type of activities have you done in the last month?

- ♥ Yelling at the TV _____ 0 point
- ♥ Walking _____ 1 point
- ♥ Swim_____ 2 points
- ♥ Work activity only _____ 3 points
- ♥ Weight lifting _____ 4 points

How often did you exercise in the last month?

- ♥ No exercise at all _____ 0 point
- ♥ Once or twice _____ 1 point
- ♥ Once or twice a week _____ 2 points
- ♥ Three or more times a week_____ 3 points
- ♥ Every day _____ 4 points

Do you hurt or ache after exercise?

- ♥ Yes _____ 0 point
- ♥ No_____ 3 points

How long do you exercise per session?

- ♥ 5 minutes or less_____ 1 point
- ♥ 5-15 minutes_____ 2 points
- ♥ 15-30 minutes_____ 3 points
- ♥ More than 30 minutes_____ 4 points

What do you do in bad weather?

- ♥ Skip exercise that day_____ 0 point
- ♥ Walk in the mall _____ 1 points
- ♥ Do calisthenics _____ 2 points
- ♥ No change in home indoor routine_____ 3 points

Score yourself:

- ♥ 0 to 5 points = please start the exercise program!
- ♥ 6 to 15 points = good start!
- ♥ 16 to 21 points = great program!

Do you have any physical limitations to exercise?

- ♥ Arthritis of knee, hip, back
- ♥ Shortness of breath during exercise
- ♥ Chest pain with exercise
- ♥ Overweight causing inability to exercise

If you have physical limitations to exercise, be careful. You may want to consider pool exercise. Read the precautions and warnings section.

<u>Food for Thought:</u>

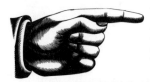 Did you know the Centers For Disease Control recommends a program of frequent moderate intensity exercise?

IT'S TIME TO SET UP YOUR EXERCISE PROGRAM!!!

Personal, Practical Program For New Athletes:

- ♥ Do something you like. If nothing comes to mind, try walking.
- ♥ If you have physical problems, try pool therapy, either water walking or water aerobics.

- Go with friends, or join an existing group.
- Do it when you feel good. If mornings are your time, plan early exercise. If you are a night owl, afternoon or early evening might be better.
- Have a little variety ready for bad days, either bad weather or bad mood.
- You can form a habit faster by doing it most every day.
- Concentrate on aerobic exercise. Your heart, your mood and your schedule will benefit most from aerobic exercise.
- Start low and go slow. You can't get into shape all at once. It takes a while!
- Stretch after exercise. It relieves muscle soreness and gets rid of lactic acid buildup. It even relaxes the mind!
- Don't get discouraged! Fine wine takes time. Your youthful vigor will return. More to the point, you will be capable of performing like you did 10-15 years ago. (Yes, this includes sexual activity.)

Food for Thought:

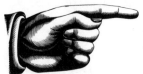 If you really want to find the time to exercise, unplug the TV. If you want to keep exercising, give away the TV.

ABOUT EXERCISE

Exercise is good for you! Remember the old saying "if you don't use it, you'll lose it?" That is the truth. Before you begin, listen to a little tale.

I'd like to take credit for motivating Maurice, but he came to see me without any prompting. Forty-five years old, he had a goal. He wanted to run the Pikes Peak Ascent race, held every August in Colorado Springs. This is no ordinary race. With an elevation gain of 8,000 feet, 14 mile distance, and variable climactic conditions, the faint of heart need not apply.

Maurice, it turned out, had made a New Year's resolution when we spoke in January. He had diabetes, high blood pressure, and high cholesterol, all mild. He was also 15 or 20 pounds overweight. After he passed his treadmill exercise test, the training began in earnest. He was smart. For a month he ran in a pool. Then as his stamina improved and the weather warmed, outdoor running commenced. Slowly and carefully, speed and distance increased.

I saw him several months later, to treat shin splints. At the same time, we checked his blood tests and weight, all of which had improved.

August came around, and I saw Maurice at the starting line. He waved and said he felt great! No, he didn't win, but I read his name in the paper. He had finished, and with a respectable time! Besides, he said, "The reasons for entering have nothing to do with winning."

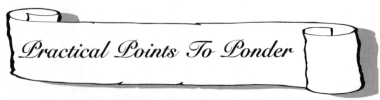

Practical Points To Ponder

EXERCISE PRESCRIPTION

- ♥ **WHY** will you exercise:
    - ◆ improve appearance
    - ◆ lose weight
    - ◆ lower blood pressure
    - ◆ improve energy
    - ◆ REVERSE HEART DISEASE
- ♥ **WHEN:** will you exercise. Dedicate the time! If you cannot decide when, it's unlikely you will start, much less stay with, your exercise. Pick a 30 minute period of the day, write it in your appointment book, and keep the appointment! Thirty minutes is 1/48th of the day.
- ♥ **TYPE:** Should be aerobic, such as walking, jogging, biking, swimming, rowing or aerobics class. Think about what you like to do. If nothing comes to mind, walk.
    - ◆ Weight lifting and bodybuilding are not very aerobic.
    - ◆ However, strength training is fine if you still have time after your aerobic exercise.
- ♥ **FREQUENCY:** Should be 5 to 6 times a week. The benefits jump enormously from two workouts to three. On the other hand, exercising seven days increases the chance of injury.
- ♥ **INTENSITY:** Should be moderate! No need to be a marathoner. Here are 3 ways to gauge this:

1. Target heart rate should be 65-85% of maximum. To calculate your maximum, take 220 minus your age. During exercise, take your pulse for 6 seconds and add a zero to find the beats per minute. See table 12 on page 191.

2. Perceived exertion, on a scale from "somewhat easy" to "very hard" should be in the moderate range, 2 or 3 steps up from "somewhat easy." See chart on following page.

3. If you cannot carry on a conversation, you are exercising too hard. If you don't even feel a little short of wind while talking, you may not be exercising hard enough.

♥ **DURATION:** Work up to 30 minutes of continuous activity. This duration is very dependent on the intensity of the activity. This does not include warm-up and cool-down.

♥ **PROGRESSION:** As you exercise, feel better, and improve your stamina, you are encouraged to progress a little at a time. However, only 10% progression per week is safe. For example, if you choose to go 10% longer, don't also go 10% harder!

Usually, people choose to speed up their activity level.

For weight loss, you may need to exercise longer.

Prior to each session, prepare by dressing in loose, comfortable clothes and athletic shoes. A 5-minute period of gentle warm-up and light stretching is advisable. This will literally warm up the muscles, make them pliant, and will prepare the heart for exertion. This also cuts down the chance of injury, and if you're injured, you can't exercise!

Following exercise, a period of slower activity should allow you to cool down. Stretch gently again. (The best stretching resource book is *Stretching* by Bob Anderson). This should leave you with the pleasant feelings of relaxation, calm, and well-being. ENJOY!

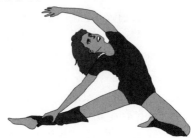

MONITORING EXERCISE INTENSITY

PERCEIVED EXERTION

Use this chart to get in, and stay in, the **moderate** range:

1. Very, very easy
2. Very easy
3. Easy
4. Average or moderate
5. Hard
6. Very hard
7. Very, very hard

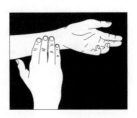

HEART RATE GUIDELINES

These are only guidelines! Exercise up to the point you feel invigorated. Don't push it to the point of feeling bad.

Age	65% of maximum heart rate	75% of maximum heart rate	85% of maximum heart rate
35	120	139	157
40	117	135	153
45	114	131	149
50	111	128	145
55	107	124	140
60	104	120	136
65	101	116	132
70	98	112	128
75	94	109	123

Table 12.

CROSS TRAINING

To keep up interest, avoid boredom, exercise different muscles, and have a contingency plan for the weather, use cross-training.

Cross training makes use of two or more different exercise methods to keep active. This also doubles your pleasure! Cross training can extend your activity level and duration. If you suffer from joint aches and pains, vary the joints you use (i.e., upper body and lower body) daily.

How fit do you want to be? Let's divide fitness into four broad categories:

- ♥ Yearning for Longevity --slow and low level
- ♥ Health Improvement--step up the pace of life
- ♥ Ready for Anything--need more variety
- ♥ Body Sculpting--lose lots of weight, keep it off, build muscles

Using cross training, I'd like to give specific examples of fitness programs you can use. I'll base them on the above categories of fitness you want to attain. If you're starting out as a couch potato (sedentary), please just do a little until you find your level of comfort.

LONGEVITY

- ♥ Move your body! Use a combination of activities.
- ♥ Monday, Wednesday, Friday take a 30-minute walk.
- ♥ Tuesday, Thursday, Saturday garden during the summer, ride a stationary bike during the bad weather.
- ♥ Sunday take off and relax.

Feel free to add in daily household chores, like climbing stairs, painting the house, moving boxes etc. to your regimen.

If bone or joint pain inhibit you, consider water exercise. This consists of swimming, walking, or exercising in a pool, in water up to the armpits. Start with 20 minutes every other day, and work up to 30 minutes 6 days a week. This is the best non-weight-bearing exercise there is, and as such helps the heart and muscles without putting undue pressure on the bones.

As you grow in strength and endurance, consider the partial weight-bearing exercises such as biking and rowing, both indoor and outdoor. If you are up to it, you can add these occasionally to change your routine. Start at 20 minutes every other day, and build up to 30 minutes 6 days a week. Integrate these new activities slowly into your routine and enjoy the variety it brings to your life!

Benefits:

This program has been proven to reduce risk of heart attack and cancer. Be prepared to wait a while untill you see the benefits--they may not be evident till the latter stages of your life. At this level of exercise, you may not turn on the endorphins or feel like the athlete in you is coming out.

HEALTH IMPROVEMENT

Let's focus on intensity. Using the three methods of gauging intensity (see exercise prescription, page 188) get to **moderate** intensity for 20 to 30 minutes, five days a week. The other two days, enjoy a relaxing walk.

To build intensity, many activities can be utilized. Brisk walking, hiking, biking, aerobics class or tapes, stair steppers, and climbing machines will do. Singles tennis, racquetball, or handball should work, but doubles probably will not.

It's true that the higher the intensity, the greater the fitness and health benefit. But this is balanced by two things: injury potential and fatigue.

There is a truism in sports science: if you are injured, you cannot exercise. However, using the cross training principle, try to alternate more intense, weight-bearing days with less intense, partial weight-bearing days. Thus some runners will run on alternate days, and swim or walk in between.

We have learned from athletes that, even when injured or sick, most can swim to hasten recovery from accident, illness or injury, without lowering their fitness level.

Benefits:

At this level, you should notice several quick results, as well as long-term benefit.

Almost immediately, you may feel more energy. Parameters such as cholesterol, blood pressure and heart rate may change. Studies prove this level of fitness wards off infection and boosts the function of the immune system. One of the best results at this level is stress reduction. A calming of mind and muscle does wonders for reducing levels of the stress hormones adrenaline and cortisone.

Long-term, dramatic reductions in heart disease and cancer rates are seen. The immune system boost may play a role in cancer reduction. HDL cholesterol levels rise to offset the buildup in the arteries. A training effect is seen on heart rate: the harder the workout over time, the lower the resting heart rate. Decline in lung function is lessened. Susceptibility to infection is reduced.

READY FOR ANYTHING

At this level, you need a combination of intensity, duration, strength, and dedication.

- From 30-60 minutes of aerobic type exercise, 5 times a week.

- Intensity in the moderate range (60% of maximum).

- Resistance exercise, such as weight training or calisthenics, 2 times a week.

- Stretching to keep the joints smooth and capable of full range of motion.

Resistance exercise is used to build bone density, strengthen and hypertrophy muscle. Far from the sweaty gyms of the past, there are many new and easier ways to get resistance exercise. (See equipment, page 197).

This is the essence of cross training. Different muscles, alternating hard and easy days, combining endurance and flexibility.

Benefits:

For those whose "athlete inside" is breaking out, the strength, flexibility and endurance necessary to engage in vigorous sports is gained. Injury avoidance is another interesting advantage at this level. This is true even in the elderly striving to reduce hip fractures. Strength and balance training has been proven to reduce falls, which consequently reduce the chance of hip fracture.

The building of a slimmer, trimmer, stronger "all American" type of physique begins at this level. Along with the body comes an enhanced ability, sexually and in sports. Your "Golden Age Olympics" participants are in this group.

Lastly, as important as the reduced risk of heart disease is, enhanced functioning of the immune system has been demonstrated. There are fewer cancers at this level of fitness--just from exercise, without any other changes in food, stress, or other risk factors.

BODY SCULPTING

Losing weight, and more important, keeping it off. Tightening and toning muscles and skin. A daunting task or an interesting challenge?

The longer and steadier the exercise duration, the longer the benefits last after the exercise ceases. Studies show that the increase in metabolism which occurs with exercise can extend 8, 10, even 12 hours afterward. So try to extend your walks to 45 minutes, or even an hour, 3 days a week. And in the spirit of cross training, add resistance training to build muscle--30 minutes twice a week. Add a swim to relieve soreness, and take the seventh day off.

For water lovers, beware! Because fat floats, swimming may be deceptively easy. Monitor the heart rate to 80% of maximum (see page 191) during 45-minute sessions, 6 days a week.

For those with joint pain, consider biking three sessions and swimming three sessions weekly. Rest the seventh day.

<u>Benefits:</u>

Long-term studies prove the only way to sustain weight loss is a daily exercise program. The easy part is losing weight, the hard part is keeping it off.

Increasing metabolism changes the energy balance. The faster the metabolism, the quicker the weight loss. As muscles grow, there is more mass to burn energy. (Our fat mass doesn't burn much energy.)

As you lose inches, the figure comes back. As weight drops, the joints feel better, as does the mood. And your risk of disease decreases--both heart disease and cancer.

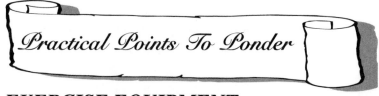

Practical Points To Ponder

EXERCISE EQUIPMENT

- ♥ Most exercise equipment, bought with the best intentions, collects dust sooner or later.
- ♥ Using exercise equipment tends to be boring. Try putting your equipment near a window, or in front of the TV, or have a stereo nearby.
- ♥ Using exercise equipment can be isolating, lonely, repetitious. There is less desire to cross train, or enjoy the great outdoors, if it's sitting in your home.
- ♥ All types of exercise equipment work--if you use them. Before spending the money, will you keep using them?
- ♥ The best equipment investment may be a pair of walking or cross training shoes!

TYPES OF EQUIPMENT

<u>Treadmills</u>:

For those who like to walk (or run) indoors. Fully weight-bearing exercise. Caution is indicated in those with leg, hip, or back problems.

Features available:

- ♥ Automatic or manual height adjustment
- ♥ Automatic speed regulator
- ♥ Computer programs, which vary from pre-programmed exercise to races and visuals

Types:

- ♥ Challenger 5.0
- ♥ Star Trac 2000
- ♥ Woodway
- ♥ Less expensive non-motorized like Jane Fonda's or Bruce Jenner's

Price: $$ to $$$$

<u>Bicycles</u>:

Many types and brands, including:

- ♥ Outdoor, mountain and road
- ♥ Indoor stationary: LifeCycle, Cybex, Randal Windracer, Schwinn Air-Dyne
- ♥ Recumbent, perhaps better for those with back problems-Diamond Back HRT by Preference

They are all partial weight-bearing, resulting in less strain than walking. It is very important to be fit properly for comfort. Most bikes have seat, length, and bar adjustments. The most critical is seat height. With the leg straight and knee locked, the heel should touch the pedal. Then start to pedal with the ball of the foot, the knee slightly bent.

Accoutrements abound. Book holders, heart rate monitors, and pedal revolution counters are a few. Several can be equipped with video monitors to play specially edited bicycle races. Race along with the pros in the Alps!

♥ The Schwinn Air-Dyne can be used with both arm and legs, making for a very hard session.

Price: varies from $$ to $$$$$

Rowing Machines:

A great aerobic workout that emphasizes the upper body. Care must be taken with form, or the back can suffer. Non weight-bearing. Can be hard on the low back.

Types:

♥ Concept II Rowing Ergometer keeps track of speed, distance, but visually doesn't catch the attention, thus can be boring.
♥ LifeRower is a little more visually pleasing, showing information on a computer screen.

Price: $$ to $$$$

Stair Steppers:

A great aerobic exercise. Very popular. A little less weight-bearing and less traumatic than running, which can be important for those with leg and back concerns.

Care must be taken to let the weight rest on the legs. There have been a variety of ailments attributed to leaning on the arms, elbows, and wrists in an effort to make the legs work faster.

Types:

♥ Stairmaster 4000 PT

♥ LifeStepper

Price: $$$ to $$$$

Cross Country Machine:

Since these machines use both the arms and legs, the exercise can be very hard. Can, however, be used with either arms or legs. No monitor or readout to hold your attention.

Types:

♥ Nordic Trak

Price: $$$ to $$$$

Resistance Trainers:

The main emphasis for your heart should be aerobic exercise. Resistance training should be reserved for those with the time, energy, and desire to supplement their aerobic exercise with strength training.

Types:

- ♥ Many types of free weights
- ♥ Rubber band resistance--Solo Flex
- ♥ Fixed weight machines--Universal or Nautilus
- ♥ Variable resistance pressure machines--Kaiser

Prices: $ to $$$$

Food for Thought:

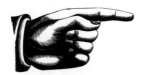

"The reasons for participating have nothing to do with winning"

A participant in the Preventive Health Institute, Danielle, had recently had a heart attack and angioplasty. She had, to her credit, also recently given up smoking!

Danielle was having a hard time with her exercise program. Never having been very active, she didn't know where to begin. And when she started walking with the group, she wheezed and was tired.

"What's wrong?" she asked during the second session. Laurin, our exercise expert, gathered enough information to conclude several things. First, Danielle didn't know how to gauge the intensity of her exercise. For her weight and level of fitness and smoking history, she was exercising too hard. After reviewing heart rate, and perceived exertion, Danielle was able to settle into a more reasonable pace.

In addition, because of inactivity, deconditioning, and smoking, Danielle was suffering from exercise-induced asthma. Every time she exercised, she wheezed. A quick trip to her doctor for a check-up and an inhaler, and Danielle made rapid progress. "I feel so much better", Danielle told us. She had just finished a 30-minute walk, keeping up with the others without shortness of breath. "Thank you."

You can even lower your blood pressure by aerobic exercise! (See figure 6)

Over 140 adults, exercising three or four days a week, for 10 to 37 weeks were studied. Exercisers averaged reductions of 6 points diastolic and 7 points systolic. This meets or exceeds the effects of most drugs used for high blood pressure (Reference 43).

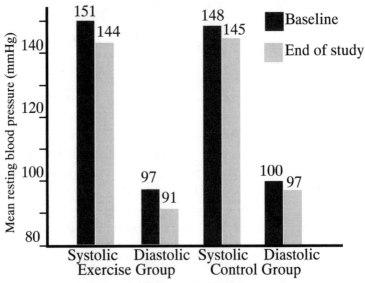

Lower your blood pressure through exercise
Figure 6. (Reference 43)

EXERCISE FOR FUN AND PROFIT

Benefits of aerobic exercise include:

- ♥ Decreased stress and blood pressure, decreased weight
- ♥ Increased HDL cholesterol, increased energy and vigor
- ♥ Reduction of deaths (see figure 7)
- ♥ Enjoyment of the freedom exercise brings

How to get started and stay moving!

- ♥ Exercise with a friend, spouse, or group
- ♥ Set a regular schedule of day, place, activity, duration
- ♥ Make it a habit, 6 days a week, with a day off for rest
- ♥ Variety is the spice of life--do more than one activity
- ♥ Use the exercise prescription as a guide
- ♥ There are now "virtual reality" exercise tapes available! As I enjoy the bike, let me tell you about a great, distracting, engaging cycling tape. The setup consists of a "wrap-around" screen which sits in front of your stationary bike. As you begin, you are a participant in the Tour de France! Up and over hills, in the pack, sprinting to the finish, you are there! Believe me, this makes your exercise session whizz by. These are available from most bike shops, and most mail order catalog stores.

How much will it cost?

- ♥ 3,500 calories in 1 pound of fat
- ♥ Decrease calories by 230 a day for 7 days = 1,610 calories
- ♥ Walk 3 m.p.h. for 30 minutes = 315 calories for 7 days = 1,890 calories
- ♥ 1,610 calories + 1,890 calories = 1 pound of fat lost each week

Precautions!

- ♥ **Chest pain:** Slow down and talk to your doctor. This symptom can go away in as little as two weeks on our program.

- ♥ **Dizziness:** during or after exercise. Dizziness has different causes. Speak to your doctor. Don't exercise when dizzy.

- ♥ **Injury:** substitute another form of exercise while recovering, i.e. swim instead of walk. Start slow and low, because an injured athlete cannot exercise effectively.

- ♥ **Hot weather:** drink plenty of fluids (bring them with you), and exercise early in the day.

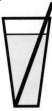

- ♥ **Cold weather:** dress in layers, cover everything, i.e. fingers, ears, nose. Consider exercising indoors. Go to an aerobics class, or use your own tape on the VCR. Use a stationary bike, stair-stepper, rowing machine, or treadmill. Be sure to play music or watch TV to distract you from the surroundings!

Myths about exercise:

- ♥ "No pain, no gain"

  Get real! Forget what the high school coach said. You should be able to appreciate the mental and physical relaxation of exercise without having to endure pain. If you do experience pain, something is wrong, and you should consult a professional.

♥ "The harder the workout, the quicker the benefits"

Especially for beginners, a hard session will cause pain, stiffness, and possible injury. For the heart, it's better to do a slower, sustained routine. Who said it had to be a "work-out." You don't have to run marathons to be an athlete. Perhaps you can call it your exercise session!

♥ "Sweating = weight loss"

Let's not confuse dehydration, which makes you feel terrible, with long-term weight (fat) loss. To prevent dehydration, always bring plenty of water. Drink every five minutes. If you wait till you feel thirsty, your body is already a quart low!

To accomplish long-term weight loss, long-term daily exercise is important. So don't get dehydrated! The best types of rhythms for weight loss are the longer, slower, moderate exertion sports. They are most efficient in burning fat, while relatively sparing the carbohydrate stores in the muscle and liver. Again, you don't have to run marathons to lose weight.

Fitness and longevity (Reference 44):

♥ Figure 7 through figure 9 show age-adjusted death rates by physical fitness categories for all-causes, for cardiovascular disease, and for cancer. Death rates show a striking decline across fitness categories in both men and women.

♥ Figure 10 illustrates the relation between fitness and all-cause mortality in men with high levels of other risk factors. Men in the moderate fitness category have much lower death rate than the low-fit men in each other risk factor group.

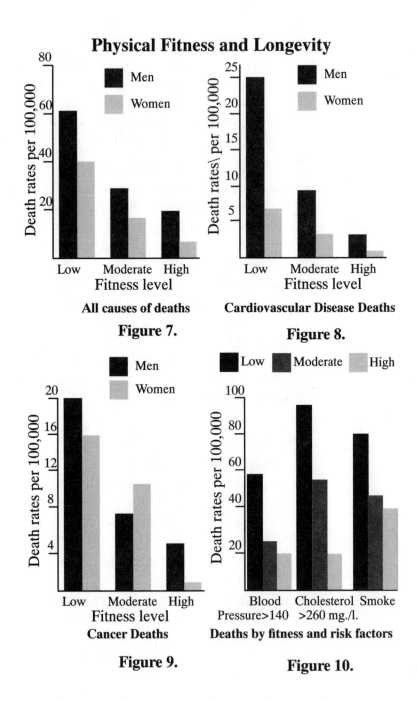

Physical Fitness and Longevity

All causes of deaths

Figure 7.

Cardiovascular Disease Deaths

Figure 8.

Cancer Deaths

Figure 9.

Deaths by fitness and risk factors

Figure 10.

WARNINGS DURING EXERCISE

SERIOUS

- ♥ _Abnormal heart action_ such as pulse becoming irregular; fluttering, jumping, or palpitations in chest or throat; sudden burst of rapid heartbeats; sudden very slow pulse when a moment before it had been on target.

  Timing can be immediate or delayed.

  Cause: Extrasystoles (extra heart beats), dropped heart beats or disorders of cardiac rhythm. This may or may not be dangerous and should be checked out by a physician.

  Remedy: Consult your physician before resuming your exercise program. Medication may temporarily eliminate the problem and allow you to safely resume exercise program; or you may have a completely harmless kind of cardiac rhythm disorder.

- ♥ _Pain or pressure in the center of the chest or the arm or throat_, precipitated by exercise or following exercise.

  Timing can be immediate or delayed.

  Cause: Possible heart pain.

  Remedy: Consult physician before resuming exercise program. Nitroglycerine may help.

- ♥ _Dizziness, light-headedness, sudden uncoordination, confusion, cold sweat, pallor, blueness, or fainting._

  Timing is immediate.

  Cause: Insufficient blood to the brain.

  Remedy: Do not take the time to cool down. Stop exercising immediately and lie down with feet elevated, or put head down between legs until symptoms pass. Consult physician before next exercise.

SELF-ADMINISTERED REMEDIES

♥ *Persistent rapid heart action near the target level even 5 to 10 minutes after exercise.*

Timing is immediate.

Cause: exercise was probably too vigorous.

Remedy: Keep heart rate at lower end of target zone. Drink fluids during exercise. If this does not help control the high recovery rate, consult physician.

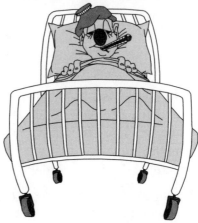

♥ *Flare-up of arthritis or gout that usually occurs in hips, knees, ankles, or big toe (weight-bearing joints).*

Timing can be immediate or delayed.

Cause: can be trauma to joints that are particularly vulnerable.

Remedy: If you are familiar with how to quiet these flare-ups of your old joint condition, use your usual remedies. Rest and do not resume exercise program until the condition subsides. Then resume exercise program with these suggestions: lower level of intensity, protective footwear, softer surfaces, try swimming or water walking. If the joint problem is new, consult a physician.

CHAPTER 10

KICK THE HABIT

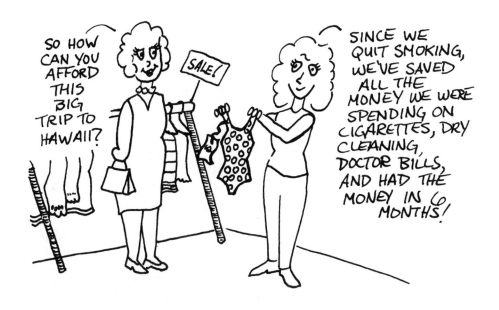

"Puff, the magic dragon, lives by the sea..."

Peter, Paul and Mary

STOP SMOKING PROGRAM

Today is the first day of the rest of your life! How long you live and how you live is to a great extent controlled by you. Nothing changes unless you agree to change. We can empower you to change, and make the process easier for you. We can save you money to boot!

Smoking negatively impacts your quality and quantity of life in many ways. It causes shortness of breath,

---

emphysema, pneumonia, wheezing, and bronchitis. It causes more heart disease than lung disease! It causes impotence, bad breath, gum disease, sinus congestion, and ulcers. Worst of all, it harms your children, and turns them into smokers.

Our program can help you! Even if you have smoked for most of your life, you can benefit from stopping. Quit, and quit now!

Think about why you smoke. It's important to know if you use smoking as a stress reducer (there are better stress reliefs), or if you are addicted (probably), or if you just have a bad habit. Once you know, there are many behavioral control strategies we can teach you.

Start the program by picking a quit day. This is the day you start to be a non-smoker. Sign the non-smoking contract! To help break the old habit, pick up a new one! Exercise helps to keep the weight down and reduce stress, but any new habit will do, as long as you do it every day.

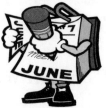

Medication is available to control the withdrawal. The nicotine patch is used daily. A drug called clonidine can help control cravings. Tricyclic, an antidepressant, when take at night can help insomnia. In higher doses, antidepressants can help the depression sometimes felt after smoking cessation. Anxiety medicine can help anxiety problems. These symptoms are common, and short term. Ask your physician about getting a prescription.

Weekly visits to your doctor are encouraged to monitor medication and your response. They also help bolster motivation, and problem solve the difficult times. Stress reduction is important, so you're not tempted to take it out on yourself by smoking.

We can help you enjoy life and feel better. Go ahead, kick the habit!! Sign on with the program, to improve your lifestyle. Take the step today, and enjoy a better tomorrow.

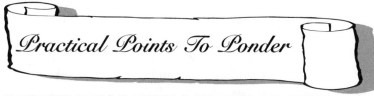

Practical Points To Ponder

DISPELLING THE MYTHS ABOUT SMOKING

Take this test on smoking, based on some of the questions we've had at the Preventive Health Institute. True or False?

♥ If you have smoked for a long time, it's not worth stopping now.

   False. Stopping now will immediately reduce your risk of heart and blood vessel disease. It also relieves shortness of breath and tendency to catch infections of the sinuses and lungs.

♥ Most smokers don't want to quit.

   False. Most smokers want to quit. Research shows 65% of smokers would like to stop.

♥ Women now are smoking less.

False. Although smoking in general has decreased, smoking among young females has **increased**.

♥ I can avoid getting fat when I quit smoking.

True. Although you will have a tendency to put on a few pounds when you quit (3 to 6 pounds), you can counteract this. An exercise program helps. So do the nicotine patches. And eating lowfat does a lot. If you do put on a few pounds, you are much better off than if you continue smoking.

♥ Older smokers find it easier to quit.

True. Men break down nicotine faster than women. Women are more likely to stick with cessation groups. For either sex, relief of symptoms such as shortness of breath, cough, and chest pain make it easier to succeed at quitting!

HOW MUCH DOES SMOKING COST?

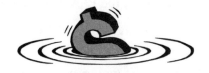

Direct Expense at $1.50 per pack:

Packs a day	Cost per Month	Cost per Year
1	$45.00	$547.50
2	$90.00	$1,095.00
3	$135.00	$1,642.50

Table 13.

Indirect Expense:

Research shows there are many indirect costs associated with smoking. Increased medical expense, lost wages due to illness, damaged clothing, furniture, carpeting, drapes, and cleaning costs amount to about $1,500 a year.

Direct Expense A Year $____ + $1,500 = $_____ Total

Could you find something else to spend the windfall on? How about a vacation? A new wardrobe?

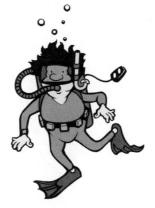

A PRACTICAL PROGRAM TO QUIT AND STAY QUIT

GET READY!

- ♥ Think about why you smoke.
- ♥ Think about how you would feel better if you quit.
- ♥ Before lighting up, ask if you really need this.
- ♥ Add up all the money you will save if you quit.
- ♥ Cut down, either the number of cigarettes or the times you smoke.

GET SET!

- ♥ Set a quit date.
- ♥ Sign a stop smoking contract. Give a copy to a loved one.
- ♥ Many smokers say cigarettes are their "friends." What or who are your "true" friends? Call or write them. Surround yourself with supportive non-smokers!
- ♥ Plan ahead. What will you do if you get the urge to smoke?
- ♥ Change your smoking routine. Do you smoke when you drink coffee? Switch to orange juice. Smoke after meals? Take a walk before clearing the table.
- ♥ When you go out, pick a smoke-free environment like a movie theatre or smoke-free restaurant. Avoid the temptation of a smoky bar.

GO!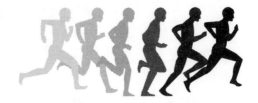

- ♥ Make an appointment with your doctor to get nicotine patches.
- ♥ The night before your quit day, throw out your cigarettes, lighters, matches, and ashtrays.
- ♥ Buy sugar free candy, gum and toothpicks. Put them where you used to keep your cigarettes.
- ♥ Dry clean your clothes.
- ♥ Take frequent walks around the block.

AFTERWARDS!

10 Things To Do Besides Smoke!

1. Don't smoke!
2. Stay away from places you used to smoke.
3. Delay when you have the urge--it will pass.
4. Take one day at a time.
5. Spend the money you save from smoking on a nice treat for yourself!

6. Enjoy a long, passionate kiss.
7. Take a hike. Besides enjoying the smell of the outdoors, your new-found lung capacity will take you places you only dreamed about before!
8. Have a discussion with a non-smoker about how good you feel.
9. Develop your (damaged) sense of smell. Put on a blindfold and identify 10 different smells. Then go to a floral shop and do the same.

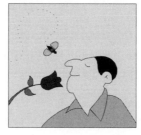

10. Put all the money you are saving in a large glass jar. Count it every day.

THE SMOKE TEST--HOW DEPENDENT ARE YOU?

If you have had a hard time quitting in the past, take this test to determine how dependent you are on smoking.

How soon after you awaken do you smoke your first cigarette?

◆ Within 30 minutes _____ 1 point
◆ After 30 minutes_____ 0 point

Do you find it difficult to refrain from smoking in places where it is forbidden (such as church, library, theatres, etc.)

◆ Yes _____ 1 point
◆ No_____ 0 point

Which cigarette would you most hate to give up?

◆ The first one in the morning_____ 1 point
◆ Any other _____ 0 point

How many cigarettes a day do you smoke?

◆ 26 or more _____ 2 points
◆ 16-25 _____ 1 point
◆ 15 or less _____ 0 point

Do you smoke more frequently during the first hours after awakening than during the rest of the day?

◆ Yes _____ 1 point
◆ No_____ 0 point

Do you smoke if you are so ill that you are in bed most of the day?

◆ Yes _____ 1 point

◆ No_____ 0 point

What is the tar content of your brand?

◆ High _____ 2 points

◆ Medium _____ 1 point

◆ Low _____ 0 point

Do you inhale?

◆ Always _____ 2 points

◆ Sometimes _____ 1 point

◆ Never _____ 0 point

Total: . . . . _____ points

SCORE:

♥ 0 - 6 = low to moderate dependence

♥ 7 - 11 = high dependence

(Reference 45)

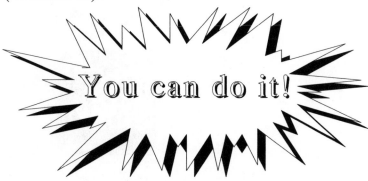

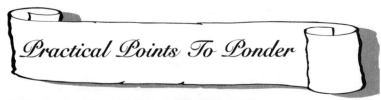

Practical Points To Ponder

YOU CAN QUIT SMOKING

♥ It takes an average of two to three tries to quit for good.

As my friend says, "opportunity only knocks 3 or 4 times!"

♥ Only you will decide if you will be a non-smoker!

♥ Fool yourself. Chew toothpicks or sugar free hard candy. Take a walk. Bite your fingernails.

♥ The urge passes! Wait, and it will leave.

♥ Give up slavery to nicotine. Be free!

♥ If you have anxiety or depression, treat it in a more healthy way.

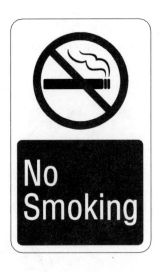

CHAPTER 11

SHOULD I BE TAKING A SUPPLEMENT??

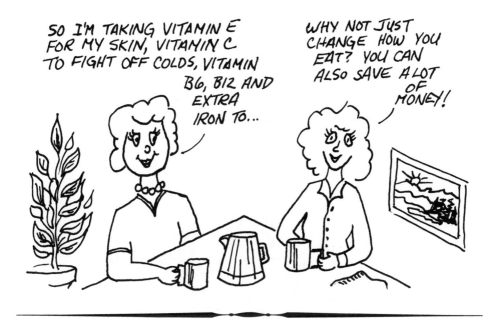

"Just a spoon full of sugar helps the medicine go down..."

Mary Poppins

Wouldn't it be great! No need to prepare food, just touch the Starship Enterprise's food synthesizer, and out pops all you need for your health. Or backpacking trips made easy. All the nourishment in pill form. Very light. Easy to prepare. Quick.

Before we get carried away, let's look at what we need and the facts about what we actually get in our food.

VITAMINS, MINERALS AND YOUR HEART

In this section, we provide an overview about nutrients and specific functions for heart health. Foods listed as sources are only those recommended on the Make the Change Food Plan. All RDA's (Recommended Dietary Allowances, 1989) listed are from the category of men, age 51 or over. RDA's for women are sometimes less.

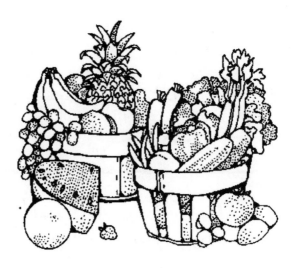

VITAMINS

♥ *Vitamin A, its precursor is beta-carotene*

RDA 5,000 IU or 1,000 µg. RE

For supplemental purposes, Beta Carotene is recommended since too much vitamin A can be toxic.

As an antioxidant, dose of beta carotene is 25 mg. or 25,000 IU.

Food item	Beta-Carotene in mg.
Sweet potato, 1/2 cup mashed	8.8
Apricots, dried, 5	6.2
Peaches, dried, 5	6.2
Carrot, raw, 1	5.7
Spinach, cooked, 1/2 cup	5.0
Cantaloupe, 1 cup	4.8
Pumpkin, cooked, 1/2 cup	3.8
Squash, winter, 1/2 cup	2.9
Tomato paste, canned, 1/2 cup	2.2
Mango, 1 cup	2.1
Beet greens, 1/2 cup	1.8
Grapefruit, 1/2	1.6
Parsley, fresh, 1/2 cup	1.6
Pepper, red, 1 whole	1.6
Broccoli, cooked, 1/2 cup	1.0

Table 14. Beta-Carotene sources

By eating plenty of fruits and vegetables, you should get all the beta-carotene you need to prevent and reverse heart disease!

♥ *Thiamin or Vitamin B$_1$*

RDA 1.2 mg. daily

Used in nervous system tissue and in carbohydrate metabolism. The need for thiamin goes up with the amount of carbohydrate in the diet.

Sources: Brewers yeast, wheat grain, whole grains and enriched cereals and breads, legumes, peas, potato, asparagus, green vegetables.

♥ *Riboflavin or Vitamin B_2*

RDA 1.4 mg. daily

Used in energy metabolism and helps convert the amino acid tryptophan to niacin.

Sources: Brewer's and baker's yeast, fortified breads and cereals, nonfat dairy products, legumes and peas, mushrooms, spinach, sweet potatoes.

♥ *Niacin or Vitamin B_3*

RDA 15 mg. daily, but when used to lower cholesterol, 1,000 to 2,000 mg. daily.

Niacin is involved in many body processes, including converting food into energy the body can use.

In high doses used for lowering cholesterol, it often causes flushing of the skin and can irritate the liver, making it necessary to monitor the liver through blood tests. Niacin should be medically supervised when taken at therapeutic high doses.

Sources: Fortified cereals, pastas and breads, whole grains and flour products, brown rice, legumes, peanuts, asparagus, green peas, corn, peaches, blackberries.

♥ *Pantothenic acid or Vitamin B_5*

Estimated safe and adequate intake; 4 to 7 mg. daily

Releases energy from carbohydrate, fat, and protein.

Sources: Nonfat dairy products, potato; white and sweet, corn, legumes and peas, nuts, avocado, broccoli, whole grain cereals, mushrooms, tomatoes.

♥ *Vitamin B_6 or pyridoxine*

RDA 2 mg. daily

Deficiency can contribute to high homocysteine levels, which increases heart disease risk when coupled with folic acid deficiency (Reference 46). Important in carbohydrate and protein metabolism and formation of hemoglobin.

Sources: Wheat germ, legumes and peas, cornmeal, quinoa, peanuts, walnuts, wheat bran, potatoes; white and sweet, enriched cereals.

♥ *Vitamin B_{12} or Cyanocobalamin*

RDA 2 µg. daily

Deficiency may cause high homocysteine levels. Deficiency also causes pernicious anemia and nerve dysfunction. Needed for energy metabolism and to make blood cells.

Sources: Fortified cereal, egg white and nonfat dairy products. Spirulina, miso, tempeh may list vitamin B_{12} on the label but they may not be reliable sources.

Strict vegetarians may want to take a vitamin B_{12} pill. Note that a micro-gram (ug) is 1000th of a gram!

♥ *Biotin*

Estimated safe and adequate intake; 30 to 100 µg. daily

Used in the synthesis of fatty acids, carbohydrate and protein metabolism. Important for the health of the circulatory system.

Sources: Yeast, nuts, soy flour, whole grains, cauliflower, peas, vegetables.

♥ *Vitamin C or ascorbic acid*

RDA 60 mg. daily; when used as an antioxidant, 1,000 mg. daily

Helps vitamin E regenerate its antioxidant effect. Less vitamin E is necessary when vitamin C is available, to prevent heart disease. Other functions include wound healing, immune system function and folic acid metabolism. Also improves absorption of iron. Deficiency causes capillary fragility and scurvy.

Sources: Guava, citrus fruits, kiwi, mango, broccoli, melon, peppers, berries, tomatoes, cabbage, potatoes.

♥ *Vitamin D or calciferol*

RDA 5 µg. daily

Controls calcium metabolism. Important along with calcium in keeping bones strong after menopause.

Produced by the skin when exposed to sunlight and found in fortified milk. People living in northern areas (or those who stay indoors) may need a supplement during winter months if they don't drink fortified milk. The skin's production of vitamin D decreases with age.

♥ *Vitamin E or alpha tocopherol*

RDA 10 mg. daily

When used as an antioxidant, 400 IU daily. (In a supplement 1 mg. = 1 IU)

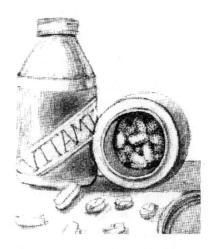

A supplement is suggested. Use the "dry" vitamin E to avoid excess oil. Proven to reduce coronary risk (Reference 47).

Food Item	Vitamin E in IU
wheat germ oil, 1 tbs.	20.3
sunflower seeds, 1 oz.	14.2
almonds, 1 oz.	6.7
cottonseed oil, 1 tbs.	4.8
safflower oil, 1 tbs.	4.6
wheat germ, 1/4 cup	4.1
peanut butter, 2 tbs.	3.0
mayonnaise, 1 tbs.	2.9
peanuts, dried, 1 oz.	2.6
mango, 1 medium	2.3

Table 15. Vitamin E content of food!

Vitamin E is often found in high-fat foods. Even if you did like wheat germ oil, the high levels of fat needed to get an antioxidant effect would be harmful.

❤ *Folic acid*

RDA 200 µg. daily

Used in cell production. Deficiency causes anemia.

Recent research shows that folic acid helps homocysteine levels stay normal to prevent atherosclerosis. There is speculation that the RDA should be raised to 400 µg. daily. As many as two out of five elderly may not get enough (Reference 48). Aim for 400 µg. daily from food sources.

Sources: Legumes and peas, green leafy vegetables, asparagus, whole wheat and fortified cereals, oranges.

♥ *Vitamin K*

RDA 80 µg. daily

One of the fat soluble vitamins which are stored in the body; others are vitamins A, D and E. Used by the liver to make the clotting proteins.

Sources: Kelp and seaweed, green tea, dark green leafy vegetables, broccoli, cauliflower, legumes and peas.

MINERALS

♥ *Calcium*

RDA 800 to 1200 mg. daily

Regulates muscle and nerve function. Important in the structure of bones. Especially important early in life, up to age 25, when the thickness of bones (bone density) builds the most. Calcium works especially well with weight-bearing exercise to build bone strength! Recent research shows supplemental calcium could reduce blood pressure in sensitive individuals

See page 155 for calcium, dairy products, and suggested daily intake.

Sources: Nonfat dairy products, figs, green leafy vegetables, broccoli, molasses, legumes, almonds. Be careful to use only fat-free milk and dairy products. Excessive protein may harm more than help, causing a net loss of calcium.

♥ *Chromium*

Estimated safe and adequate intake; 50 to 200 µg. daily.

A trace mineral that helps insulin work more efficiently. Low intake may be associated with high blood cholesterol levels and increased risk of heart disease (Reference 49). It is thought that many Americans have substandard intakes because of highly processed diets. Diabetics may benefit from a supplement or higher intake from food.

Sources: Brewer's yeast, whole grain foods, orange juice.

♥ *Copper*

Estimated safe and adequate intake: 1.5-3 mg. daily.

Important in helping maintain healthy arteries, blood cells and blood vessels. Low intakes have been related to increased blood cholesterol in some studies. Also helps iron absorption (Reference 50).

Sources: Whole grain breads and cereals, nuts, dried beans and peas, dark green leafy vegetables.

♥ *Iron*

RDA varies according to age and sex

Iron is important in transporting oxygen throughout the bloodstream. Deficiency causes anemia which is more common in premenopausal women and children. High levels could increase risk of heart disease, apparently by oxidizing LDL. Absorption of iron is inhibited by calcium-- in dairy products and supplements; also by tea and fiber.

Sources: Tofu, legumes and peas, dried fruit, molasses.

♥ *Manganese*

Estimated safe and adequate intake; 2 to 5 mg. daily

Assists in enzyme actions in body. Deficiency causes ringing in the ears and muscle weakness.

Sources: Whole grain breads and cereals, legumes, green leafy vegetables.

♥ *Magnesium*

RDA 350 mg. daily

Important for nerve function, muscle action, and may lower blood pressure. Implicated at deficiency levels in cardiac arrhythmias. Therefore, very important if the heart is stressed to have adequate levels.

Sources: Nuts, legumes, green leafy vegetables and whole grain cereals.

♥ *Selenium*

RDA 70 μg. daily; as an aid to the antioxidant vitamins, up to 200 μg. daily.

Some studies show low blood levels of selenium are related to increased risk of heart disease and some types of cancer.

Sources: Brazil nuts, cashews, kidney beans, mushrooms and onions. Also found in many vegetables, depending on how fertile the soil grown in is.

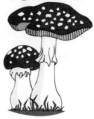

♥ *Zinc*

RDA 15 mg. daily

Important for immune system function, wound healing, reproductive health and taste buds. Deficiency causes inability to make sperm.

Sourcee: Wheat germ, miso, dried beans and peas, yeast.

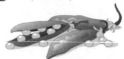

PHYTOCHEMICALS: Not an artificial additive, but natural plant chemicals! There are thousands of these naturally occurring compounds in food which may not be in pills! Many are probably yet to be discovered. ONE REASON TO BE CAREFUL WITH SUPPLEMENTS: they may give you false assurance that your diet has all the nutrients it needs from a pill. However, if you don't eat whole foods in sufficient quantity, you miss out on all the benefits of phytochemicals. They are not available in pill form! The evidence is mounting that they are very useful to your health!

Here are just a few phytochemicals that we know about:

Limonene: (citrus fruits) Helps produce enzymes that may dispose of potential carcinogens.

Allyl sulfides: (garlic, onions, leeks, and chives) Increase the production of glutathione S-transferase, which may make carcinogens easier to excrete.

Dithiolthiones: (broccoli) Help form glutathione S-transferase and may block carcinogens from damaging a cell's DNA. Yes, even though President Bush hated it, broccoli is good for you!

Ellagic acid: (grapes, apples) Scavenges carcinogens and may prevent them from altering a cell's DNA.

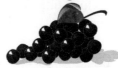

Protease inhibitors: (soybeans, dried beans) Suppresses the production of enzymes in cancer cells, which may slow growth.

Caffeic acid: (grapes and other fruits) Speeds the production of enzymes that make carcinogens more water soluble, which may aid in ridding them from the body.

Ferulic acid (fennel) Binds to nitrates in the stomach, which may prevent conversion to carcinogenic nitrosamines.

Phytic acid: (grains) Binds to iron, which may prevent the release of "free radicals." These free radicals may oxidize LDL to form the "bad, bad cholesterol."

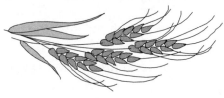

Isothiocyanates: (bok choy, broccoli, brussels sprouts, cabbage, cauliflower, collards, kale, kohlrabi, mustard greens, rutabaga, turnip greens, and turnips) Trigger the formation of glutathione S-transferase, which blocks carcinogens from damaging a cell's DNA.

Indoles: (soy protein) Stimulate enzymes that make estrogen less effective, which could reduce the risk of breast cancer.

Phytosterols: (soy) Slows down the reproduction of cells in the large intestine, which may prevent colon cancer (like high fiber content).

Isoflavones: (soy) Blocks the entry of estrogen into cells, which may reduce the risk of breast or ovarian cancer. Pharmaceutical trials (Nolvodex) are underway to investigate this same mechanism to block breast cancer. May also lower cholesterol and increase HDL.

ARTIFICIAL COLORS AND PRESERVATIVES

No known benefit (besides extending shelf life). Some may be harmful. Common reactions include:

- Allergy, as in asthma, hives, swelling, runny nose.
- Headaches
- Rashes

<u>A partial list of additives:</u> (There are many more!)

- BHT, BHA
- Monosodium glutamate (Accent)
- Salt (common table salt)
- Benzoates (sodium benzoate)
- Sulfiting agents (sodium metabisulfate used in restaurants)
- Tartrazine (FD&C Yellow No. 5)
- Antibiotics (found in meat and chicken)
- Hormones (found in beef)
- Nitrites and nitrates (found in hot dogs & lunch meats)
- Saccharin and aspartame (sweeteners)

For those of you wishing to minimize risk, organically grown food has the lowest levels of additives.

To keep the risks in perspective, however, please know that by eating more fruits and vegetables, you can lower your risk of heart disease and cancer. Washing produce well (or using products like FIT) can help if you worry about pesticides.

As we now know, by eating less meat, chicken, fish, and dairy we can also lower our risk of heart disease and cancer!

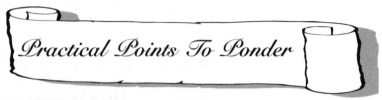

Practical Points To Ponder

NUTRIENTS

- ♥ Supplement vitamin E with 400 IU of "dry" E. Some selected groups may need extra vitamins. Special circumstances such as osteoporosis, and anemia may require higher levels, and a supplement.

- ♥ Fruit, vegetables, and grains have natural chemicals, many of which are protective against disease!!!!!

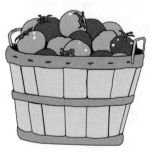

- ♥ Mega dosing and supplements don't make up for a poor choice of foods (what you don't eat **may** hurt you)!

- ♥ Meat has a lot of harmful things in it! For your health, eat a lot more fruits, vegetables, whole grains and legumes (beans and peas).

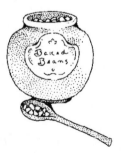

CHAPTER 12

PHARMACEUTICALS

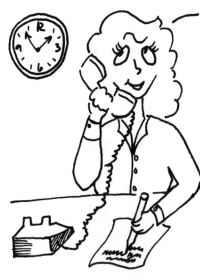

SO DOCTOR, IF THERE AREN'T ANY DRUGS TO MAKE ME THIN, HOW ABOUT SOMETHING TO MAKE ME RICH?...NO?...LUCKY? ...NO?...FUNNY?...NO... ANYTHING THAT WILL REDUCE MY TAXES?... PAINT MY HOUSE?... CLEAN THE OVEN?... MOW THE LAWN?... HOW ABOUT...

"Double, Double, toil and trouble. Fire burn and cauldron bubble."

William Shakespeare
Mac Beth

DRUG THERAPY

A patient of mine, Henry, was raking his yard. He started to suffer from excruciating chest pains. Rescue 911 was called, arrived quickly, and determined he was having a major heart attack! He was transported to the hospital.

The decision upon arrival quickly became whether to treat with a "clot busting" drug to dissolve a blood clot blocking the artery saving heart muscle from damage. The risk of bleeding, especially of cerebral hemorrhage, was thought to be 3 or 4%. Henry's heart attack was very serious; it might very well be fatal. Of the several clot-busting drugs, he was given t-pa.

Henry had very good results. His potentially fatal heart attack was turned into a very small one. He went home in 3 days, feeling much improved. Good outcome, no side effects.

When he visited his cardiologist, Henry brought along a copy of his hospital bill. "Why does this t-pa cost so much! I think $1,200 a dose is excessive. Aren't there any alternatives?" As it turns out, Henry found that streptokinase is available for about 40 to 50% of the price of t-pa. For first time use, it works about as well. It has about the same rate of side effects as t-pa. And the experts are divided equally on the question of which drug is "better."

The makers of t-pa had, however, just finished a major advertising campaign. National journals carried their ads; touting t-pa as superior, worth the money. And low and behold, sales went up. Coincidence, or change in usual practice based on sound scientific research?

Henry told his cardiologist, "If I ever again have to have a clot-busting drug, please use streptokinase. I don't have money to burn!"

Henry had been sensitized to this issue in the past. He had suffered side effects from two other heart drugs. He stopped one of them, without informing his doctor. With the other, he simply reduced the dose to reduce the side effects. Unfortunately for Henry, it was a bad move for his heart.

FACTORS IN DRUG THERAPY

Compliance and adherence

The former term is older. Now most studies use the friendlier term "adherence" to describe how people take their prescriptions. Adherence drops the more frequently a drug is supposed to be taken.

Many people don't take their prescriptions as prescribed:

- ♥ Daily: 80 to 90%
- ♥ Twice a day: 60 to 75%
- ♥ Three times a day: 40 to 50%
- ♥ Four times a day: 27 to 30%

Out of a ten-day antibiotic prescription, most people only take seven to eight days worth!

Drug taking also varies by the type of condition:

- ♥ Arthritis: 70%
- ♥ Epilepsy: 50%
- ♥ Diabetes: 50%
- ♥ Hypertension: 40%

Costs

Generic drugs usually cost 25 to 50% less than brand name or "proprietary" drugs. It's easy to spend $100 a month or more per drug. The drug companies want to recoup the expenses of research, development, and advertising. Generic companies don't have as much overhead. Generics are held to a slightly less strict standard by the FDA regulations. For some drugs, this is a cause for concern.

"Why am I taking this drug?"

Research shows that 60% of patients do not know why a particular medication has been prescribed.

Side effects, i.e., benefit vs. risks

In most situations, the **benefit** is relatively small. A 50% reduction may mean a difference from 8% to 4%. In other situations, such as my patient with the heart attack, the benefits may be much greater.

Risks of drugs include allergy, nausea, fatigue, failure of the drug to work for the condition or disease, and drug interactions (with food or with other drugs).

As with everything in medicine, a detailed weighing of the risks versus benefits should be discussed by both doctor and patient prior to prescribing any therapy. Don't forget to ask about alternatives to the drug!

"I want to do it on my own!"

Some people, because of past experiences or anecdotal stories, are afraid or unwilling to take any drug. Others are unrealistic, in that they wish to be better, but will not make the necessary changes to ensure they will make themselves well.

"I forgot"--the passive way to refuse

For any drug to have an effect, the patient <u>has</u> to believe in the need for the medication, and must take it as directed! Please, if you feel you cannot take a prescription for any reason, inform your physician!

A final caution on drug interactions

For those on more than one drug, the possibility of interactions between drugs increases greatly. There may be:

♥ Failure of the drug to work

♥ Potentiation of the drug's action

♥ Diminution of the action

♥ Damage to liver, kidney, or other body system

Why the emphasis on drugs?

♥ Pharmaceutical manufacturers drive (i.e. fund) the research studies. Being one of the largest multi-national industries, the companies are constantly on the look out for new products, and new uses for old ones.

For example, the acne drug, Retin-A, was developed many years ago to treat teen-age acne. Sales were moderate. It had a niche, however, and the company continued marketing. About four years ago, a research dermatologist studied its effects on age-related and sun-related wrinkling. After publication of the findings, the general news media picked up the story. Soon sales of Retin-A skyrocketed! Profits surpassed all records, mostly because the **price went up** as the popularity rose.

- Drugs are profitable.
- Pharmacology is taught in medical school.
- It is the tradition of allopathic physicians to treat the disease, not the person (don't assign blame). The idea of personal responsibility for health is not stressed in medical schools.
- It's "easier" to take a pill than to make lifestyle changes. Taking a pill doesn't require much effort, and requires no change in habits.
- People are not aware of the power they possess through diet, exercise and stress reduction to influence their disease. They feel helpless in the face of both the disease and the medical system.

WASTE AND DUPLICATION IN THE INDUSTRY

The case of the "me-too" drugs. Me-too drugs start as useful, big selling drugs for one company. Then, other companies come up with similar drugs, designed for the same condition, and promote heavily, hoping for a "big winner."

Prices vary, sometimes tremendously, within each class. Efficacy, or usefulness, can also vary, but to a much smaller degree.

Cardiovascular drugs:
- Anti-hypertensives, over 40
- Cholesterol lowering: Mevacor and Zocor (same company), Pravachol, Lescol
- Diuretics or water pills

Antidepressants:
- ❤ Prozac
- ❤ Zolof
- ❤ Paxil
- ❤ Effexor

Antibiotics:
- ❤ Cephalosporins
  First Generation - Cefalexin
  2nd Generation - Cefactor
  3rd Generation - Cefuroxime

WHAT WILL COMPANIES DO TO SELL THE PRODUCT?

David Kessler M.D., head of the Food and Drug Administration, recently wrote on this subject (Reference 51).

- ❤ Too many "me-too" drugs are developed and marketed.
- ❤ Companies put on "seeding trials" which appear to serve no scientific purpose. They pay doctors to prescribe their drug.

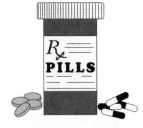

- ❤ Promotional materials may use false and misleading claims of superiority over a competing drug.
- ❤ Many companies, health insurance agencies, and agents try to get patients switched from their original prescriptions to "me-too" drugs marketed by their companies.

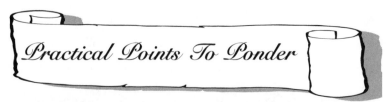

Practical Points To Ponder

HELPING MEDICATIONS HELP YOU

- ♥ Form an alliance with your doctor. Let you doctor help you be well.

- ♥ If you don't intend to take a medication, tell your doctor. Hopefully, you will be ready to start the lifestyle changes necessary to make yourself well.

- ♥ If you are having side effects, tell your doctor.

- ♥ Ask if there are alternatives that are less expensive, and have fewer side effects, than the treatment being prescribed.

- ♥ Don't take anything unless you understand what it is for and is supposed to do.

- ♥ If you take more than one drug, make sure they don't interact with each other. Ask your physician under what conditions you should take the drug:

  - ♦ Full or empty stomach
  - ♦ Time of day
  - ♦ Mixed with or apart from other drugs
  - ♦ Precautions such as sunlight exposure
  - ♦ How long to take the drug
  - ♦ What to do about side effects

THERE IS MORE THAN ONE WAY TO ACHIEVE YOUR GOALS. IF YOU HAVE QUESTIONS OR RESERVATIONS, WORK WITH THE EXPERTS TO MAKE A SUITABLE PLAN!

CHAPTER 13

A WORD ON CANCER PREVENTION

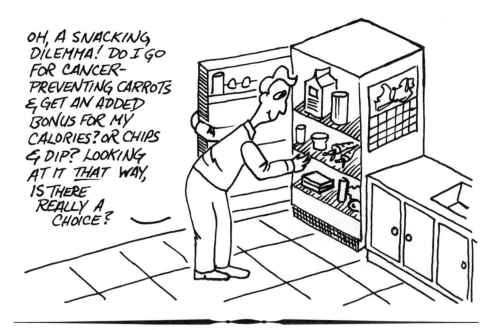

OH, A SNACKING DILEMMA! DO I GO FOR CANCER-PREVENTING CARROTS & GET AN ADDED BONUS FOR MY CALORIES? OR CHIPS & DIP? LOOKING AT IT THAT WAY, IS THERE REALLY A CHOICE?

"The fear factor."

The fear factor affects many of us, like it did "Miss Nancy" the teacher. She was paralyzed by the fear of cancer, even after she noted the blood in the toilet.

"It's just hemorrhoids!" she said when I explained I need to take a look. It was an epic conversation, extending not only through that visit, but through two months. Finally, she consented to the examination, which showed a colon cancer. She wanted surgery to "get it out, all out." She didn't

---

want to hear the surgeon talk about possible spread to the liver.

By great good fortune, "Miss Nancy" had a localized cancer, cured by surgery. She is alive and well today.

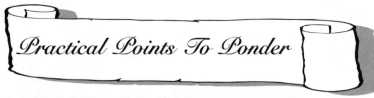

Practical Points To Ponder

DISPROVING CANCER MYTHS

Today is your lucky day! The day we disprove myths and misconceptions surrounding cancer, such as:

"Doesn't **everything** cause cancer?" and

"There is nothing **I** can do to reduce my risk."

- ♥ All the factors used in this book to prevent and reverse heart disease will help prevent cancer!
- ♥ The leading cause of cancer is smoking.
- ♥ The next leading cause of cancer is SAD, the Standard American Diet.
- ♥ Other important causes are heavy alcohol use and sunlight.
- ♥ The fear factor is present in us all. Don't let it paralyze you! The facts and statistics tell us that cancer is a preventable, treatable, and in many cases a curable disease.

NATIONAL CANCER INSTITUTE NEWS

♥ Smoking contributes to cancers of:

lung	mouth	larynx
esophagus	pancreas	bladder
kidney	stomach	uterus and cervix

♥ 35% of cancers are related to what we eat. These cancers include:

colon	breast	prostate
stomach	liver	ovary
lining of the uterus (endometrium)		

♥ Americans eat too much fat. Populations with a high-fat diet have a high incidence of colon, breast, and prostate cancer.

♥ Alcohol--heavy drinking (over 2 drinks of alcohol per day) is associated with cancers of the:

mouth	throat	esophagus
liver		

THE CASE FOR LIFESTYLE AND CANCER PREVENTION

There are four life-style elements that are associated with reduced cancer risk. The good news is that by following the Make the Change Eating Plan, you will automatically be improving most of these areas. Remember the 4 F's:

♥ **Fat intake:** A high fat intake is generally related to higher cancer risk. Also, several studies have linked saturated fat intake with higher risk for lung and breast cancer (reference 52). Our program automatically cuts the fat and saturated fat in your diet to almost 0!

♥ **Fiber Intake:** Insoluble fiber, the type found in whole grains and cereals, fruits and vegetables, is associated with a decreased risk in cancer rates, especially of the colon. Recommended fiber intake is 20 to 30 grams per day. (The average intake in the U.S. is 5 to 10 grams) See the following table 16.

Food	Grams of fiber
All bran cereal, 1/4 cup	10 to 13
Wheat bran, 1/4 cup	7
Raisin bran, 3/4 cup	5
Bulgur, 1/2 cup	3
Figs, 3	7
Prunes, 3	5
Blackberries or raspberries, 1/2 cup	5
Dates, 5	4
Pear with skin, 1	4
Orange, 1	3
Spinach, 1/2 cup drained	6
Corn, 1/2 cup	5
Broccoli, 1/2 cup	4
Sweet or white potato, 1/2 cup	4
Whole artichoke	4

Table 16. Fiber content of food

♥ **Phytochemicals:** Vegetarians are generally healthier than their meat-eating counterparts for several reasons. Their diets are lower in fat, animal protein, saturated fat and cholesterol, but their diets are also chock-full of whole grains, fruits and vegetables.

Research shows that people who eat more fruits and vegetable have a reduced cancer risk. Why? There are thousands of "phytochemicals" or plant chemicals in food that are biologically active. Beta-carotene is just one of many compounds called carotenoids, that may **all** be helpful in keeping cancer away. Right now, there is only one way to get these compounds in your diet--by eating lots of fruits, vegetables, whole grains and beans. There is a lengthier discussion of phytochemicals and soy foods in Chapter 4.

♥ **Fitness:** The more fit have much reduced rates of cancer. See figure 11 below and reference 44.

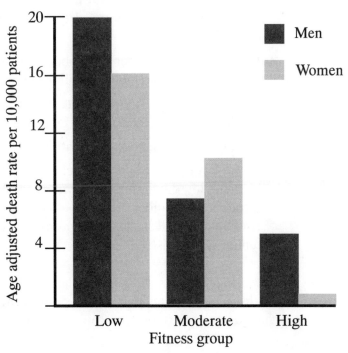

The Effect of Exercise on Cancer Prevention

Figure 11.

CASE BY CASE CANCER PREVENTION

Cancer is the second leading cause of death in the USA.

♥ Lung cancer is the most common cancer among both sexes. Clearly, women have caught up to men in lung cancer deaths, due in large part to intense advertising by the tobacco industry.

PREVENTION: Do not smoke. Quit now if you do smoke. (Chapter 10)

♥ In women, breast cancer is number 2 in deaths.

PREVENTION: Since breast cancer has been linked to a high-fat diet, cut way down on fat (reference 53). There is some evidence that an eating plan high in antioxidants, especially beta-carotene, also prevents this cancer. (Page 224)

♥ In men, prostate cancer is number 2. It has been said that if you live long enough, you will develop prostate cancer.

PREVENTION: Since prostate cancer has been linked to a high-fat diet, cut down on fat (reference 54).

♥ Colon cancer is next on the death list for both sexes.

PREVENTION: Since colon cancer has been linked to a high-fat, low-fiber diet, cut down on fat. In addition, those on a high-fiber diet have a reduced colon cancer risk. Take in at least 25 to 30 grams of fiber every day to reduce cancer risk (reference 55).

These four cancers account for the vast majority of cancer deaths. They can all potentially be prevented. You cannot change your genes, but you can control your habits.

CHAPTER 14

DELIGHTFUL, DELICIOUS, DELECTABLE RECIPES

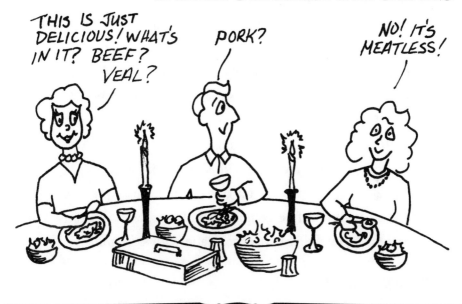

"One cannot think well, love well, sleep well, if one has not dined well."

Virginia Woolf

WHAT YOU WILL FIND

BREAKFAST IDEAS

- Lowfat pancakes with fresh berries
- Fat-free cereal with skim milk, yogurt or soy milk, toast and juice
- Egg Beater omelette with mushrooms, green pepper and fat-free cheese
- Toasted bagel with fat-free cream cheese, jam and cappucino
- Very Berry Shake (page 316), raisin toast
- Zucchini Bread (page 263) with fat-free cream cheese, fresh melon
- Pumpkin Muffins (page 261), oatmeal with cinnamon sugar
- Toasted fat-free pound cake with strawberries, hot cocoa
- Cereal with skim milk, fresh fruit, toast
- Grape nuts cooked in microwave with skim milk and dates
- Lowfat waffles with strawberry fat-free cream cheese spread and berries
- Fat-free yogurt with fat-free granola, cantaloupe, toast
- Crepes (page 287) with fresh peaches, latte with skim milk

LUNCHES ON THE GO

Listed below are some good choices for 2 favorite quick meals--frozen meals and cup of soups. Of course, leftovers also make good quick lunches as do sandwiches made of bean spreads, leftover tofu loaf or veggie burgers.

Frozen meals:

Please keep in mind that these meals are made for people trying to lose weight--most are 200-300 calories. **This is not enough for an entire meal for most people!** Add fresh fruit, salad, some type of bread and skim milk or yogurt, and dessert if desired.

The following meatless meals have 6 grams of fat or less. Sodium is enclosed in brackets:

Lean Cuisine:

 Macaroni and cheese with broccoli [460 mg.]
 Angel hair pasta with vegetables and marinara sauce [420 mg.]

Weight Watcher's:

 Garden Lasagna [540 mg.]
 Fettucini Alfredo with Broccoli [540 mg.]

Smart Ones:

 Lasagna Florentine [590 mg.]
 Ravioli Florentine [420 mg.]

Celentano's:

 Broccoli Stuffed Shells [520 mg.]

Healthy Choice:

 Garden Potato Casserole [520 mg.]
 Macaroni and Cheese [580 mg.]
 Pasta Shells Marinara [390 mg.]
 Cheese Ravioli Parmigiana [290 mg.]

Michelina's:

 Spaghetti Marinara [680 mg.]

Lowfat Cup-of-Soups--the New Rage for a Quick Meal:

Add a salad, fruit, crackers and you've got a tasty, filling, high fiber meal!

Varieties that have 1.5 grams of fat or less and less than 500 mg. sodium include: Taste Adventure Minestrone, Casbah La Fiesta, Nile Spice Lentil Home Style, Nile Spice Chili n' Beans, Fantastic Foods Jumpin' Black

Bean, Fantastic Foods Leapin' Lentil Over Couscous, Fantastic Foods Splittin' Peas, Spice Hunter Kasbah Curry and Nile Spice Red Beans and Rice. (source: Supermarket Savvy Fact Sheet, © 1994, Leni Reed Associates)

FIFTEEN MINUTES MEALS

Some of these menus incorporate recipes from Make the Change--page number in parentheses; others use frozen or convenience foods.

- Tossed salad
- Pasta E. Fagiol (page 296)
- Fresh fruit

- Broccoli coleslaw
- Sloppy Joes (page 298)
- Fresh mango or canned peaches

- Tomatoes in balsamic vinegar
- Tortillas with steamed vegetables and Dijon Sauce (page 277)
- Yogurt with strawberries

- Fiesta Pasta Salad (page 271)
- Baked tortilla chips with fat-free bean dip
- Fresh fruit salad

- Green Giant Create a Meal, Sweet and Sour Vegetables cooked with tofu

- Vanilla pudding

- Health Valley Fat-Free Chilli
- Tossed salad with fat-free cheese
- Frozen banana with fig bars

- Hash browns (found near eggs) with Roasted Red Pepper Sauce (page 279)
- Steamed frozen vegetable mix
- Bush's vegetarian baked beans
- Fat-free cookies and skim milk

- Leftover Pasta With Quick Alfredo Sauce (page 297)
- Steamed vegetables
- Sorbet

- Bean and Rice Burritos (page 281)

- Jello with fruit

- Minute Minestrone (page 267)
- Boursin Cheese Spread (page 256) on crusty french bread
- Fresh apple

- White kidney beans, cucumber, tomato, lettuce, sprouts and green onions in fat-free vinaigrette inside pita bread
- Very Berry Shake (page 316)

- Hoppin' John (page 292)
- Coleslaw with fat-free Ranch dressing
- Fat-free cookies

- Veggie burger on bun with sauteed onion and mushrooms
- Hash browns
- Fresh melon

- Tomatoes and cucumbers in fat-free vinaigrette
- Black bean tostadas (canned fat-free refried beans on baked corn tortilla)
- Healthy Choice Lowfat Ice Cream

- Three bean salad
- Bulgur and Veggie Mix (page 305)
- Frozen yogurt with blueberries

- Instant couscous with chick peas, mixed vegetables and Curry Sauce (page 276)
- Pita bread
- Microwave baked apple

- Tossed Salad
- Pita pizza (pita bread topped with fat-free cheese, pizza sauce, veggies)
- Mango sorbet

- Fresh carrots and broccoli with fat-free dip
- Creamy spinach burritos (see Delightful Spinach page 306)
- Mixed fruit salad

- Green Giant Create a Meal Vegetable Lo Mein with tofu or black beans
- Berries and Fat-free Pound Cake

- Grilled vegetables (Eggplant, squash, onions) on french bread with marinara sauce or fat-free cream cheese
- Fat-free hot fudge sundae

A MONTH OF DINNER MENUS

- Baby salad mix
- Spring Vegetables With Cream Sauce Over Angel Hair Pasta (page 300)
- Fresh fruit, cookies
- French bread

- Oriental Salad (page 273)
- Broccoli and Tofu Stir Fry (page 284)
- Steamed rice
- Fruit sorbet

- Black Bean And Corn Salad (page 270)
- Greek Pilaf (page 307)
- Delightful Spinach (page 306)
- Melon balls

- Coleslaw with fat-free slaw dressing
- Boston Baked Beans (page 283)

- Bulgur and Veggie Mix (page 305)
- Healthy Choice Cookies n' Cream Lowfat Ice Cream

- Leek and Potato Soup (page 265)
- Happy Family Dinner (page 291)
- Angel food cake with fresh fruit and 2 Tbs. Cool Whip light

---

- Romaine lettuce salad
- Ratatouille (page 309) with bow tie pasta
- Strawberry sorbet

- Grated Celery Root in Vinaigrette (page 275)
- Lentil Soup (page 266) garnished with tomatoes and fat-free sour cream
- Crusty sourdough bread
- Strawberry Tiramisu (page 314)

- Raw vegetables with fat-free dip
- Baked tortilla chips with fat-free salsa
- Colorado Stuffed Peppers (page 286)
- Easy Blueberry Cobbler (page 313)

- Jicama and Orange Salad (page 272)
- Oat Nut Burgers (page 295) on wheat buns with all the trimmings
- Oven Fried Potatoes (page 308)
- Fat-free vanilla pudding with bananas

———◆———

- Grated Carrots with Fat-Free Vinaigrette (page 275)
- Spinach Stuffed Shells (page 299)
- Steamed yellow squash
- Healthy Choice Bordeaux Cherry Chocolate Chip Lowfat Ice Cream

———◆———

- Lowfat vegetable soup
- Crustless Quiche (page 289)
- Greek Pilaf (page 307)
- Hard rolls
- Fat-free cookies

———◆———

- Aspen Black Bean Soup (page 264)
- Steamed mixed vegetables
- Roasted new potatoes
- Fresh fruit

———◆———

- Summer Vegetable Salad with Very Green Dressing (page 274)
- Tofu Loaf (page 302)
- Wild rice
- Fat-free frozen yogurt topped with warmed lite apple pie filling

———◆———

- Romaine, boston and curly endive salad
- Vegetarian Chili (page 269) with Baked tortilla chips
- Chili N' Cheese Cornbread (page 260)
- Fresh raspberries topped with fat-free vanilla yogurt

———◆———

- Minute Minestrone (page 267)
- Pasta with marinara sauce
- Steamed broccoli
- Fresh fruit

———◆———

- Spinach salad with boiled egg white mushrooms and toasted walnuts
- Spaghetti with Lentil Spaghetti Sauce (page 278)
- Stuffed "Med" Bread (page 262)
- Raspberry sorbet

———◆———

Make The Change For A Healthy Heart   **253**

- Minute Minestrone Soup (page 267)
- Vegetable Lasagna (page 303)
- Easy Peach Cobbler (page 313)

———————

- Vegetable Salad with Very Green Dressing (page 274)
- Millet Burgers with Garlic Mushrooms (page 293)
- Healthy Choice Lowfat Mint Chocolate Chip Ice Cream

———————

- Mushroom and Barley Soup (page 268)
- Tofu Loaf with tricolored grilled peppers (page 302)
- Fresh fruit salad

———————

- Tossed salad
- Vegetarian Pizza
- Chocolate Almond Dream (page 312)

———————

- Coleslaw with Marzetti's Fat-Free Slaw Dressing
- Vegetarian Chili (page 269)
- Entenmann's fat-free pound cake with strawberries

———————

- Black Bean, Corn and Barley Salad (page 270)

- Cheese Enchiladas (page 285)
- Fat-free hot fudge sundae

———————

- Raw vegetables with fat-free Ranch dressing
- Stuffed Eggplant Creole (page 301)
- Bananas foster (page 310)

———————

- Oven Fried Zucchini (page 259)
- Pasta with quick alfredo sauce (page 297)
- Tiramisu (page 314)

———————

- Mexican Artichoke dip with Pita crisps (page 258)
- Bean and Rice Burritos (page 281)
- Fresh fruit salad with yogurt

———————

- Baked potato
- Steamed mixed vegetables
- Lima beans with fat-free sour cream
- Fresh berry mix

———————

- Tossed salad
- Bean and Cornbread Bake (page 280)
- Watermelon

———————

- Sliced tomatoes with fresh basil and vinaigrette
- Spring vegetables with cream sauce wrapped in tortillas
- Waldorf salad made with fat-free mayonnaise

———————◆•◆———————

- Broccoli & cauliflower salad

- Rigatoni with Lentil Spaghetti Sauce (page 278)
- Fresh orange

———————◆•◆———————

- Grated Carrots in Vinaigrette (page 275)
- Mock Egg Foo Young
- Brown rice
- Easy Peach Cobbler (page 313)

ABOUT THE MAKE THE CHANGE RECIPES

The goal of the recipes included here is to get you started with healthy eating. There are many other great lowfat and vegetarian cookbooks to go to from here--they are listed under Suggested Reading (page 330). We tried to give you some familiar recipes, like lasagna, that have been modified. In addition, we've included some items that are new to you to broaden your horizon of eating. We tried to keep it practical, so you won't find any recipes that take all day to cook. Many recipes call for canned and convenience items to cut your time in the kitchen.

For almost all recipes you will need nonstick cooking spray like Pam--keep plenty on hand. To cut the sodium in recipes, use no salt added tomato products. Rinsing other canned products will also cut the sodium.

Where a range of an ingredient is indicated, the lesser was used to analyze the recipe. (as in 1 to 2 tsp. salt). Fiber content is listed when 3 grams or more. Enjoy!

BOURSIN CHEESE SPREAD

This recipe is from More Lowfat Favorites by Ceacy Thatcher. Try it with pita bread crisps, crackers, raw vegetables, or in crepes with veggies.

Yield: 12-1/4 cup servings

    8 oz. fat-free margarine
    16 oz. fat-free cream cheese
    2 cloves fresh garlic minced or 1 tsp. chopped garlic in jar
    1/2 tsp. leaf oregano
    1/4 tsp. leaf marjoram
    1/4 tsp. leaf thyme
    1/4 tsp. leaf basil
    1/4 tsp. dill weed
    1/4 tsp. white pepper

Preparation:

1. Using a hand mixer or spoon, mix all ingredients until well blended.
2. Chill one hour before serving.

Nutrient Analysis per Serving:

- ♥ 40 calories
- ♥ 0.7 gram fat
- ♥ 5 grams protein
- ♥ 2.6 grams carbohydrate
- ♥ 373 mg. sodium

CAJUN GARBANZO NUTS

This is a great substitute for nuts and are good on a salad as well.

Yield: 4-1/3 cup servings

Ingredients:

1-15$^1/_2$ oz. can garbanzo beans
1 tsp. cajun spice mix or spice mix you prefer
Cooking spray

Preparation:

1. Preheat oven to 325°.

2. Drain and rinse beans.

3. Spread beans close together on baking sheet.

4. Sprinkle 1/2 of spice mix over beans. Lay hands on top of beans and gently roll. Sprinkle remaining spice on.

5. Bake 45 to 55 minutes, testing often at the end of baking time to find the texture you prefer. Baking longer will produce a texture similar to corn nuts. Baking shorter will produce softer texture in the middle, chewy on the outside.

Nutrient Analysis per Serving:

- ♥ 83 calories
- ♥ 1.5 grams fat
- ♥ 4 grams protein
- ♥ 14 grams carbohydrate
- ♥ 4 grams fiber
- ♥ 338 mg. sodium

MEXICAN ARTICHOKE DIP

When company calls, this is a quick recipe to throw together!

<u>Yield</u>: 10-1/4 cup servings

Ingredients:

2/3 cup fat-free mayonnaise
1/3 cup parmesan cheese, freshly grated
1/4 tsp. hot pepper sauce
1/2 tsp. garlic powder
1 cup soft bread crumbs
2-14 oz. can artichoke hearts, drained and chopped
1-4 oz. can green chiles, your choice of hotness!
(for really mild tastebuds, use 1/2 can)

Preparation:

1. Preheat oven to 350°. Combine first 5 ingredients. Gently fold in artichokes and green chiles.

2. Spray a 1 quart casserole dish with cooking spray. Spoon dip mixture into dish and bake 20 minutes. Or microwave on MEDIUM for 12 to 14 minutes.

3. Serve with baked pita bread triangles, fat-free corn chips or crackers.

Nutritional Analysis per Serving:

- ♥ 59 calories
- ♥ 1.1 grams fat
- ♥ 3 grams protein
- ♥ 9 grams carbohydrate
- ♥ 334 mg. sodium

OVEN FRIED ZUCCHINI STICKS

<u>**Yield:**</u> 48 sticks, 4 servings

<u>**Ingredients:**</u>

1/2 cup Italian bread crumbs
2 Tb. fat-free parmesan cheese
1/4 tsp. garlic powder
3 medium zucchini
Water
1 cup fat-free or lowfat spaghetti sauce

<u>**Preparation:**</u>

1. Preheat oven to 475°. Spray cookie sheet with cooking spray.

2. Place bread crumbs, cheese and garlic powder in a zip-lock bag; shake well to combine. Set aside.

3. Cut each zucchini lengthwise into 8 pieces; cut each piece in half lengthwise. Fill a saucer with water. Dip each zucchini stick in water and drop into bag of crumb mixture. Shake until coated on all sides and place on cookie sheet. Repeat with rest of sticks.

4. Bake for 10 to 15 minutes or until brown and tender. Serve with warm spaghetti sauce.

<u>**Nutrient Analysis per Serving:**</u>

- ♥ 94 calories
- ♥ 1.2 grams fat
- ♥ 5 grams protein
- ♥ 17 grams carbohydrate
- ♥ 437 mg. sodium

CHILE N'CHEESE CORNBREAD

<u>**Yield:**</u> 6 pieces

<u>**Ingredients:**</u>

1 package Gold Medal Golden Cornbread & Muffin Mix
1/3 cup skim milk
2 egg whites
2 Tbs. water
2 Tbs. dry butter buds
1 Tbs. (or more if you like) drained green chiles
1 clove or 1/2 tsp. chopped garlic
1/2 cup drained whole kernel corn
1/2 cup fat-free grated cheddar cheese
Cooking spray

<u>**Preparation:**</u>

1. Preheat oven to 425°. Blend all except last 2 ingredients in bowl until just mixed. Gently stir in corn and cheese.

2. Pour into 8 inch round or square pan that has been sprayed with cooking spray. Sprinkle grated cheese on top. Bake 10 to 14 minutes.

<u>**Nutrient Analysis per Serving:**</u>

- ♥ 135 calories
- ♥ 1.3 grams fat
- ♥ 4 grams protein
- ♥ 28 grams carbohydrate
- ♥ 296 mg. sodium

PUMPKIN MUFFINS

Yield: 12 muffins

Ingredients:

2 egg whites
1 Tbs. tub margarine
1/2 cup raisins (optional)
2 tsp. baking powder
1/2 tsp. salt
1/2 tsp. each ground cinnamon
and nutmeg

2/3 cup brown sugar
3/4 cup skim milk
2 cups all-purpose flour
1/2 tsp. baking soda
1/4 tsp. ground ginger
3/4 cup + 2 Tbs. canned unsweetened
pumpkin

Preparation:

1. Preheat oven to 400°. In large bowl, combine egg white, margarine, pumpkin, sugar and milk. In small bowl combine remaining ingredients. Fold wet and dry ingredients together until just blended. Fold in optional raisins.

2. Spray loaf pan with cooking spray. Pour batter into pan and bake for 20 to 25 minutes. Remove from pan and cool on wire rack.

Serving suggestion:

Serve with Orange Cream Cheese Spread: Mix fat free cream cheese, orange marmalade and powdered sugar to taste.

Nutritional Analysis per Serving:

- ♥ 169 calories
- ♥ 4 grams protein
- ♥ 1.3 grams fat
- ♥ 214 mg. sodium

STUFFED "MED" BREAD

This bread is a wonderful accompaniment with soup, salad or Mediterranean dish.

Yield: 5-2$^1/_2$ inch slices

Ingredients:

1 package Pillsbury Crusty French Loaf (found with canned biscuits)
1/2 medium sized eggplant   8 sun dried tomato pieces
1/4 cup each water and red wine   1/4 tsp. salt
1 clove garlic   1/2 tsp. basil
1/4 tsp. oregano

Preparation:

1. Preheat oven to 350°. Spray cookie sheet with cooking spray.

2. Boil water and wine together. Remove from heat and add tomatoes. Let sit several minutes until soft and hydrated.

3. Peel eggplant. Slice into 1/2 inch slices; cut each slice into 6 to 8 pieces.

4. Spray nonstick saute pan with cooking spray. Add garlic and cook 1 to 2 minutes. Add eggplant and herbs and cook 5 minutes. Add tomato sauce and tomatoes; stir and cover. Cook 5 to 10 minutes until eggplant is tender.

5. Open french loaf can and unroll loaf. Spoon eggplant mixture onto dough and spread out to within 1 inch of edge of dough. Roll up like a jelly roll and tuck each end of bread under. Place on cookie sheet.

6. Bake for 30 to 35 minutes. Cool on wire rack 5 minutes before slicing.

Nutrient Analysis per Serving:

♥ 170 calories   ♥ 33 grams carbohydrate

♥ 1.2 grams fat   ♥ 448 mg. sodium

♥ 6.7 grams protein

ZUCCHINI BREAD

You won't believe it's fat-free! Make two and freeze one!

Yield: 1 loaf, 12 slices

Ingredients:

$1^1/_2$ cups flour

1/2 tsp. ground nutmeg

1/2 tsp. baking powder

1 package of butter buds

3/4 cup sugar

1/4 cup applesauce

1/2 tsp. vanilla

1/2 cup grape nuts (optional)

1 tsp. cinnamon

1/2 tsp. baking soda

1/4 tsp. salt

2 egg whites

1/2 cup skim milk

1/4 tsp. dried grated orange rind

1 cup zucchini, unpeeled and grated

Preparation:

1. Preheat oven to 350°. Spray loaf pan with cooking spray.

2. Sift flour, cinnamon, nutmeg, soda, baking powder and salt. Add Butter Buds to mixture; set aside.

3. Mix egg whites, sugar, orange rind, milk and vanilla.

4. Add sifted ingredients and blend in grated zucchini. Add grape nuts if desired.

5. Pour into loaf pan and bake 60 to 70 minutes.

Nutrient analysis per Serving:

♥ 113 calories

♥ 0.2 gram fat

♥ 2.6 grams protein

♥ 26 grams carbohydrate

♥ 108 mg. sodium

ASPEN BLACK BEAN SOUP

A hearty, delicious soup that is great after a morning walk.

Yield: 6-1$^1/_3$ cups servings

Ingredients:

1 medium onion, chopped	1 tsp. dried whole oregano
3 cloves garlic or 3 tsp. chopped garlic in jar	2-15 oz. cans black beans, drained and rinsed or 3 cups
1/2 tsp. dried whole thyme	1/2 tsp. cumin
1/4 tsp. cayenne pepper	3 cups fat-free chicken broth
2 tomatoes, chopped	1/2 cup onion, chopped finely

1/2 cup fat-free grated mozzarella or cheddar cheese (optional)

Preparation:

1. Spray skillet with cooking spray. Cook onion and garlic until tender, about 5 minutes, add water if needed. Stir in spices, cook 2 to 3 minutes.

2. Place 1/2 of beans in blender and puree until smooth, adding broth as needed to help make smooth.

3. Add pureed beans, remaining broth and beans to onion mixture. Bring to boil and then lower to MEDIUM heat and simmer 20 to 30 minutes.

4. Serve garnished with diced tomatoes, onions and cheese.

Serving suggestion:

For a complete meal, add a salad, and cornbread or a grilled vegetable sandwich.

Nutritional Analysis per Serving:

- ♥ 144 calories
- ♥ 8.4 grams protein
- ♥ 449 mg. sodium
- ♥ 1.3 grams fat
- ♥ 26 grams carbohydrate
- ♥ 8 grams fiber

LEEK AND POTATO SOUP

Yield: 16 servings

Ingredients:

2 lbs. of leeks
4 medium carrots
8 potatoes
2 cups evaporated skim milk
Salt & pepper to taste

Preparation:

1. Peel potatoes and carrots. Cut leeks down the center and rinse thoroughly. Cut all vegetables into 1 inch pieces.

2. Place all vegetables into large pot of hot water. Bring to a boil and simmer, covered for 45 minutes, or until potatoes and carrots are tender. Since carrots take longer, you may start them off first in the pot.

3. Drain 90% of the water off. Puree in batches in blender with small amounts of milk in each batch.

4. Place all pureed soup back in large pot. Stir well, adding additional milk if needed.

Nutrient Analysis per Serving:

- ♥ 141 calories
- ♥ 0.3 gram fat
- ♥ 6 grams protein
- ♥ 30 grams carbohydrate
- ♥ 75 mg. sodium (with no salt added)

LENTIL SOUP

Yield: 6-1$^1/_2$ cups servings

Ingredients:

1 pound dry lentils	7 cups water
1 cup fat-free chicken broth	1 to 2 tsp. salt
6 large crushed garlic cloves	2 medium onions, chopped
2 stalks celery, chopped	2 to 3 medium carrots, sliced
1/2 tsp. basil	1$^1/_2$ tsp. thyme and oregano
1 bay leaf	

Red wine vinegar, and chopped tomatoes to garnish on top
Lots of freshly ground black pepper

Preparation:

1. Brown onions, garlic, and celery in a pan sprayed with cooking spray, adding 1 Tbs. of water as needed.

2. Place lentils, herbs, water, and salt in a kettle. Bring to a boil, lower heat to a very slow simmer, and cook covered, for 20 to 30 minutes.

3. Add black pepper and carrots. Cover, and let simmer another 30 to 45 minutes, stirring occasionally.

4. Remove bay leaf. Serve hot, with a sprinkle of red wine vinegar and chopped tomatoes on top of each bowlful.

Nutritional Analysis per Serving:

- ♥ 182 calories
- ♥ 0.7 gram fat
- ♥ 13 grams protein
- ♥ 33 grams carbohydrate
- ♥ 612 mg. sodium
- ♥ 9 grams fiber

MINUTE MINESTRONE SOUP

Yield: 4-1$^1/_2$ cups servings

Ingredients:

5 oz. frozen spinach, thawed
1-8 oz. can tomato sauce
1-14$^1/_2$ oz. can diced tomatoes
1 cup green beans
1 cup cooked pasta
1-14 oz. can kidney beans, drained
1 tsp. dried or 2 Tbs. fresh minced parsley

1 medium carrot, diced
1/2 tsp. onion powder
1/2 tsp. garlic powder
1 tsp. Italian seasoning
1/2 tsp. dried basil

Preparation:

1. Combine all ingredients in a 1$^1/_2$ quart saucepan.

2. Simmer 10 to 15 minutes or until carrots are tender. Add more water for a thinner soup.

Variation:

Omit green beans and carrots and add a 10 oz. package frozen mixed vegetables, adding more water if necessary.

Nutrient Analysis per Serving:

- ♥ 189 calories
- ♥ 2.1 grams fat
- ♥ 9 grams protein
- ♥ 38 grams carbohydrate
- ♥ 980 mg. sodium
- ♥ 8 grams fiber

MUSHROOM AND BARLEY SOUP

<u>**Yield:**</u> 6-1$^1/_2$ cups servings

<u>Ingredients:</u>

1/2 cup uncooked pearl barley	4$^1/_2$ cups water
1 medium onion, chopped	3 cups fat-free chicken broth
2 medium cloves garlic, minced	1 lb. mushrooms, sliced
3 to 4 Tbs. dry sherry	Freshly ground black pepper

<u>Preparation:</u>

1. Place the barley and 1$^1/_2$ cups of the water in a large saucepan. Bring to a boil, cover, and simmer until the barley is tender (20 to 30 minutes).

2. Meanwhile, heat 1 to 2 Tbs. of water in a skillet. Add the onions and saute for about 5 minutes over MEDIUM heat; add garlic and mushrooms. Cover and cook, stirring occasionally, until everything is very tender, about 10 to 12 minutes.

3. Add the saute with all its liquid to the cooked barley, along with the remaining 2 cups of water and 3 cups of broth. Grind in a generous amount of black pepper, and simmer, partially covered, another 20 minutes over very LOW heat. Season to taste, and serve.

<u>Nutritional Analysis per Serving:</u>

- ♥ 97 calories
- ♥ 0.4 gram fat
- ♥ 3.3 grams protein
- ♥ 18 grams carbohydrate
- ♥ 348 mg. sodium
- ♥ 3 grams fiber

VEGETARIAN CHILI

Yield: 6-1$^1/_2$ cups servings

Ingredients:

2-15 oz. cans kidney beans, drained
1-28 oz. can crushed tomatoes in puree
1-15 oz. can tomato sauce   1/4 cup uncooked bulgur wheat
1 medium onion, chopped   2 large clove garlic, minced
2 to 4 tsp. chili powder   2 tsp. cumin
1/2 tsp. oregano
1 medium zucchini or 1 medium bell pepper, chopped
Finely minced parsley, tomato and onion for topping
Cayenne pepper or pepper to taste

Preparation:

1. Heat a small amount of water in a nonstick pot. Add onion and garlic. Saute over MEDIUM heat about 5 to 10 minutes, add zucchini or bell pepper, and saute until all the vegetables are tender.

2. Add the tomatoes, tomato sauce, beans, spices and bulgur. Simmer over lowest heat, stirring occasionally, for 15 minutes. Taste to adjust seasonings, and serve hot, topped with parsley, chopped fresh tomato and onion if desired.

Serving Suggestions:

🍎 Over baked tortilla chips with fat-free cheddar cheese stirred in

🍎 Rolled up in a flour tortilla

🍎 Stuffed in a bell pepper

Nutritional Analysis per Serving:

♥ 220 calories   ♥ 1.0 gram fat

♥ 12 grams protein   ♥ 44 grams carbohydrate

♥ 1056 mg. sodium   ♥ 11 grams fiber

BLACK BEAN AND CORN SALAD WITH TORTILLA CHIPS

<u>Yield:</u> 4-1 cup servings

<u>Ingredients:</u>

1-16 oz. can black beans, drained and rinsed
1 cup corn, drained
1/2 cup fat-free Italian dressing
1/2 cup plain nonfat yogurt
1/2 tsp. cumin
1/8 tsp. garlic powder
2 tomatoes, quartered
2 cups romaine lettuce, torn
2 Tbs. fat-free cheddar cheese (optional)

<u>Preparation:</u>

1. Mix corn, beans and dressing. Marinate in refrigerator at least 30 minutes. Mix yogurt and spices. Add pepper to taste. Set aside

2. Spoon bean mixture over lettuce. Top with yogurt sauce or serve on the side. Garnish with tomato quarters and tortilla chips.

<u>Variation:</u> Add 1/2 cup cooked barley and 1 to 2 Tbs. additional dressing to corn and black bean mixture.

<u>Serving Suggestion:</u> Serve with baked tortilla chips or make your own by cutting corn tortillas into quarters, spray with cooking spray and sprinkle with spices. Bake at 375° until crispy, turning once.

<u>Nutritional Analysis per Serving</u>

- ♥ 155 calories
- ♥ 7.8 grams protein
- ♥ 289 mg. sodium
- ♥ 0.81 gram fat
- ♥ 30 grams carbohydrate
- ♥ 8 grams fiber

FIESTA PASTA SALAD

This is a Shirley Lippincott's recipe for a great quick meal and a good way to use leftover pasta and vegetables. Besides the pasta and vegetables, you can be creative! Throw in whatever you have in the refrigerator or pantry.

Yield: 4-2$^1/_2$ cups servings

Ingredients:

> 1 pound bag of frozen "Fiesta Style" Vegetables
> 4 cups cooked pasta (rotini or wheels work nicely)
> 1-14 oz. can artichoke hearts, drained, quartered
> 1 large tomato, cut in chunks
> 1-15 oz. can beans, your choice
> 1$^1/_2$ cups fat-free salad dressing

Preparation:

1. Thaw vegetables for several hours or run warm water over to thaw.
2. Mix pasta, vegetables and all ingredients. Mix gently until blended.
3. For best taste, refrigerate for at least 30 minutes to let flavors blend.

Nutritional Analysis per Serving:

♥ 344 calories

♥ 1.6 grams fat

♥ 13 grams protein

♥ 67 grams carbohydrate

♥ 312 mg. sodium

♥ 10 grams fiber

JICAMA AND ORANGE SALAD

Yield: 4-3/4 cup servings

Ingredients:

2 navel oranges, peeled, sectioned and cut in two;
   or 1 can mandarin orange segments, drained and rinsed
2 cups jicama, jullienne-cut
3 Tbs. orange juice
2 Tbs. rice vinegar
Leaf lettuce

Preparation:

1. Combine oranges and jicama in a bowl.
2. Mix together juice and vinegar. Toss lightly with orange mixture.
3. Chill before serving. Serve over lettuce leaf.

Nutritional Analysis per Serving:

- 93 calories
- 2 grams protein
- 0.1 gram fat
- 3 mg. sodium
- 2.5 grams fiber

ORIENTAL SALAD

<u>**Yield:**</u> 4-1$^1/_2$ cups servings

<u>**Ingredients:**</u>

4 cups shredded romaine lettuce
1 celery stalk, finely chopped
1 to 2 green onions, sliced
1/2 cup sliced water chestnuts, rinsed
1-10 oz. package frozen snow peas, thawed or steamed and cooled
1 teaspoon sesame seeds
1/2 cup mung bean sprouts
1-11 oz. can mandarin oranges (optional)

DRESSING

<u>**Ingredients:**</u>

3/4 cup white wine vinegar
1/4 cup sugar
1/2 tsp. sesame oil
1 tsp. soy sauce
1/4 tsp. pepper

<u>**Preparation:**</u>

1. Toss salad ingredients. Mix together dressing and toss with salad.

<u>**Nutrient analysis per Serving:**</u>

- ♥ 85 calories
- ♥ 1.1 grams fat
- ♥ 2 grams protein
- ♥ 19 grams carbohydrate
- ♥ 102 mg. Sodium

SUMMER VEGETABLE SALAD

Ingredients: Pick a mixture of vegetables from below to suit your taste. Use about 1 to $1^1/_2$ cups total vegetables per person.

Sprouts	Carrots	Celery
Broccoli	Cauliflower	Beets
Cabbage (green and red)	Spinach	Green beans
Bell peppers (all colors)	Zucchini	Yellow squash
Cucumber	Snow peas	Red onion
Scallions	Radishes	Fresh herbs
Tomatoes and mushroom slices as toppings		

Preparation:

1. Peel when necessary; mince or grate everything and mix well.

VERY GREEN DRESSING

Yield: 4-1/3 cup servings

Ingredients:

1 Tbs. chopped, packed parsley   5 medium-large fresh spinach leaves
1 cup 1% or fat-free buttermilk   1 medium clove garlic
1/2 tsp. salt   1 tsp. lemon juice
1/4 cup fat-free sour cream   12 medium fresh basil leaves
1/2 of a small zucchini, cut in chunks

Preparation:

1. Puree all ingredients in a blender or food processor and mix with salad.

Nutritional Analysis per Serving--vegetables and dressing:

- ♥ 80 calories
- ♥ 0.9 gram fat
- ♥ 5 grams protein
- ♥ 14 grams carbohydrate
- ♥ 375 mg. sodium
- ♥ 3 grams fiber

VEGETABLES IN VINAIGRETTE

It is a french tradition to have grated vegetables in vinaigrette as a starting course.

Yield: 4 servings

Ingredients:

Use the following amounts of one or more vegetables:

    7 finely grated carrots
    1/2 finely grated celery root
       (now available in the U.S., also called celeriac)
    2 thinly sliced cucumbers
    1/3 head finely grated red cabbage

Add:

    1/2 cup fat-free vinaigrette (strong flavored best)
    1/4 cup finely chopped parsley
    Salt and pepper to taste

Preparation:

1. Combine all ingredients. Let marinate at least 30 minutes.
2. For a variation, add 1 to 2 Tbs. fat-free sour cream to vinaigrette.

Nutritional Analysis per Serving:

- ♥ 30 calories
- ♥ 0.1 gram fat
- ♥ 0.5 gram protein
- ♥ 7.3 grams carbohydrate
- ♥ 51 mg. sodium

CURRY SAUCE

Yield: 6-1/4 cup servings

Ingredients:

10 oz. silken lowfat tofu
1/4 cup skim milk
1 to 2 tsp. curry powder
1/2 tsp. salt
Pepper to taste

1 to 2 cloves garlic, minced
1/2 tsp. cumin
1 Tbs. ketchup
1/4 tsp. Garam Masala

Preparation:

1. Blend all in blender. Heat over stovetop or in microvewave until warmed through.

Note: Garam Masala is a spice blend found in gourmet shops and large health food stores. If not found, you can replace with 2 pinches of cinnamon, 1 pinch of ground cardamom, and 1 pinch of ground cloves.

Serving suggestions:

1. Serve over rice or vegetables, or as topping on crepes.
2. Try with a mixture of cauliflower, peas, and potatoes.
3. Spinach or eggplant.
4. Potatoes, peas, green beans.
5. Lentils and tomatoes.

Nutritional Analysis per Serving:

- ♥ 21 calories
- ♥ 0.6 gram fat
- ♥ 3.5 grams protein
- ♥ 0.8 gram carbohydrate
- ♥ 225 mg. sodium

DIJON SAUCE

Yield: 4-1/4 cup servings

Ingredients:

1/2 cup fat-free sour cream
1/2 cup plain nonfat yogurt
1 to 2 Tbs. Dijon style mustard
Salt, pepper and garlic powder to taste

Preparation:

1. Mix all ingredients. Heat until just warm--do not boil.

Serving Suggestions:

Great over vegetables, for a dipping sauce for fresh artichokes, over crepes, or with roasted or baked potatoes.

Nutritional Analysis per Serving:

- 43 calories
- 0.1 gram fat
- 2.5 grams protein
- 66 mg. sodium

LENTIL SPAGHETTI SAUCE

Yield: 8-1 cup servings

Ingredients:

1 medium onion, chopped	1 green pepper, chopped
5 cloves garlic, minced	3 cups fat-free beef broth
$1^1/_2$ cups water	1-1 lb. bag dry lentils
$2^3/_4$ tsp. Italian seasoning	1/2 tsp. onion powder
1/2 tsp. salt	1 Tbs. vinegar

1/2 to 1 tsp. crushed red pepper flakes
1-28 oz. can no added salt stewed tomatoes
2-15 oz. cans low sodium tomato sauce
Freshly ground pepper to taste

Preparation:

1. Spray a dutch oven with cooking spray. Add, onion, pepper and garlic. Saute over MEDIUM heat until tender, adding 1 to 2 Tbs. of water as necessary.

2. Add broth, lentils, red pepper and Italian seasoning. Bring to a boil. Cover, reduce heat and simmer 45 to 60 minutes, until lentils are tender.

3. Stir in tomatoes and vinegar. Bring to a boil, reduce heat and simmer 30 minutes or until desired consistency is obtained. Stir often.

Leftover Idea: Puree some leftover sauce in blender and you have Lentil Sloppy Joes! You may need to add additional tomato sauce to taste.

Nutritional Analysis per Serving:

- ♥ 270 calories
- ♥ 0.9 gram fat
- ♥ 18 grams protein
- ♥ 49 grams carbohydrate
- ♥ 826 mg. sodium
- ♥ 7 grams fiber

ROASTED RED PEPPER SAUCE

<u>Yield</u>: 5-1/3 cup servings

<u>Ingredients:</u>

    1/2 green onion, chopped
    1/4 tsp. garlic powder
    1 heaping cup roasted red peppers (can be bought in a jar)
    2 Tbs. white wine vinegar (can be flavored)
    1/3 cup fresh parsley, torn into pieces
    1/3 cup nonfat yogurt or fat-free sour cream

<u>Preparation:</u>

1. Puree all ingredients except yogurt in food processor. Place in micro-wave safe dish and cook on MEDIUM-HIGH for 2 minutes.

2. Fold in yogurt or sour cream. Heat another 30 seconds on HIGH. Serve with vegetables, over vegetable crepes, veggie burgers or grilled tofu.

<u>Nutritional Analysis per Serving:</u>

- 25 calories
- 0.1 gram fat
- 1 gram protein
- 5 grams carbohydrate
- 16 mg. sodium

BEAN AND CORNBREAD BAKE

Yield: 4 servings

Ingredients:

3 cups cooked or canned beans
  (pinto, black beans, kidney beans or any combination will work.)
1/3 cup each: chopped green pepper, celery and onion
2 Tbs. ketchup
8 oz. tomato sauce
1 tsp. dry mustard
1/4 tsp. pepper
1 package Gold Medal Corn Muffin Mix
2 Tbs. honey
2 egg whites
1/3 cup skim milk
1/4 cup grated fat free cheddar cheese (optional)

Preparation:

1. Spray pan with cooking spray. Add pepper, celery and onion with 1 to 2 tablespoons water and cook until tender. Add beans, tomato sauce, ketchup, dry mustard and pepper.

2. Mix cornbread mix with honey, egg white and milk. Stir until just blended. Fold in cheese, if desired.

3. Spray 2 quart baking dish with cooking spray. Add beans and top with cornbread batter. Bake 30 to 35 minutes until bread is golden brown.

Nutritional Analysis per Serving:

- ♥ 471 calories
- ♥ 2.7 grams fat
- ♥ 21 grams protein
- ♥ 95 grams carbohydrate
- ♥ 814 mg. sodium
- ♥ 7 grams fiber

BEAN AND RICE BURRITOS

Yield: 6 servings

Ingredients:

12 small reduced fat flour tortillas
3 cups cooked brown rice
2-16 oz. cans flavored refried beans
 (such as Rosarita's Zesty Salsa Fat-Free Refried Beans)
Cumin, chili powder, cayenne pepper to taste
1 head romaine lettuce, shredded
3 to 4 scallions, chopped
2 ripe tomatoes, chopped
Oil and fat-free Mexican salsa

Preparation:

1. Preheat oven to 350°. Wrap tortillas, 6 each, in aluminum foil, sprinkling with a few drops of water before wrapping up. Bake 10 to 15 minutes. (Tortillas can also be warmed in microwave for 2 to 3 minutes but become tougher)

2. Put beans and cooked rice in a saucepan. Add more spices to taste. Heat 5 to 10 minutes. Meanwhile, prepare the vegetables.

3. Place bean mixture down the middle of each tortilla. Top with lettuce, scallions, tomato, and salsa. Tuck in the top and bottom edges, roll into a burrito, and serve immediately, topped with additional salsa to taste.

Nutritional Analysis per Serving:

- ♥ 440 calories
- ♥ 4.6 grams fat
- ♥ 15 grams protein
- ♥ 87 grams carbohydrate
- ♥ 11 grams fiber

BLACK BEAN ENCHILADA CASSEROLE

This quick and easy casserole was modified from Janet Boyd's recipe.

<u>**Yield:**</u> 4 servings

<u>**Ingredients:**</u>

    1-15 oz. can Southwestern style Black Beans (with spices), undrained
    1-15 oz. can Del Monte Chili Style Tomatoes
    1/4 cup picante sauce
    3 corn tortillas
    4-6 oz. fat free cheese

<u>**Preparation:**</u>

1. Preheat oven to 350°. In bowl, mix beans, tomatoes and sauce. Spray 2 quart round casserole dish with cooking spray.

2. Place 1 corn tortilla in bottom of dish. Add 1/3 of bean mixture, 1/3 of cheese, another tortilla, 1/3 of bean mixture, another tortilla and rest of bean mixture.

3. Bake 20 minutes. Sprinkle remaining 2 Tbs. cheese on during last 5 minutes of cooking.

4. To make this recipe in a 9 x 13 pan, use 3 cans of black beans and 3 cans of tomatoes and 12 tortillas, overlapping 6 tortillas on each layer.

<u>**Low sodium variation:**</u>

Cook 1 sliced onion, 1 tsp. chopped garlic and 1 sliced bell pepper until tender. Add 15 oz. can stewed tomatoes and 3/4 cup picante sauce. Use $1^1/_2$ cups cooked black beans with $1^1/_2$ tsp. cumin and 1 tsp. chili powder.

<u>**Nutritional Analysis per Serving:**</u>

- 250 calories
- 1.7 grams fat
- 1211 mg. sodium
- 20 grams protein
- 39 grams carbohydrate
- 10 grams fiber

BOSTON BAKED BEANS

Yield: 6-1$^1/_4$ cups servings

Ingredients:

5 cups cooked white beans or
    pinto beans
1 medium onion, chopped
2 Tbs. maple syrup
1 Tbs. soy sauce
1$^1/_2$ tsp. dry mustard
1/2 tsp. ground cinnamon
3 to 4 Tbs. molasses

2 medium sized, tart apples,
    peeled and cut into small chunks
1-16 oz. can tomatoes, chopped
1 Tbs. vinegar
1 Tbs. parsley flakes
1$^1/_4$ tsp. powdered ginger
1/4 tsp. black pepper

Preparation:

1. Saute the onion in a small amount of water, until soft. Add the remaining ingredients, except for the beans. Cook and stir for about 5 minutes.

2. Preheat oven to 350°. Stir beans into mixture, and transfer to a deep casserole or a 9 x 13 inch baking pan. Cover tightly with foil, and bake for 30 to 45 minutes.

3. Serve warm with rice, cornbread, or warmed tortillas.

Nutritional Analysis per Serving:

- ♥ 272 calories
- ♥ 1.2 grams fat
- ♥ 13 grams protein
- ♥ 322 mg. sodium
- ♥ 10 grams fiber

BROCCOLI AND TOFU STIR FRY

<u>**Yield:**</u> 4-1$^1/_2$ cups servings

<u>**Ingredients:**</u>

2 Tbs. chicken broth
2 tsp. grated fresh ginger
3 cloves garlic, minced
3 green onions, chopped
3 cups chopped fresh broccoli
1 Tbs. vinegar
1 Tbs. hoisin sauce
2 Tbs. reduced sodium soy sauce
1/4 cup water
1 lb. firm tofu, crumbled into smaller than bite size pieces

<u>**Preparation:**</u>

1. Heat chicken broth in a non-stick pan. Add ginger, garlic and green onions. Saute 2 minutes. Add broccoli and stir fry until broccoli is tender crisp. Add more chicken broth or water to pan if necessary.

2. Mix together vinegar, hoisin sauce, soy sauce and water. Set aside. Add tofu to broccoli and stir fry 2 more minutes. Add sauce mixture and continue cooking until warmed through.

3. Serve over brown rice, bulgur or noodles.

<u>**Nutritional Analysis per Serving:**</u>

- ♥ 117 calories
- ♥ 2.48 grams fat
- ♥ 15 grams protein
- ♥ 11 grams carbohydrate
- ♥ 383 mg. sodium
- ♥ 3 grams fiber

CHEESE ENCHILADAS

This recipe is from More Lowfat Favorites by Ceacy Thatcher.

<u>**Yield:**</u> 12 enchiladas

<u>**Ingredients:**</u>

    1-15 oz. can no salt added tomato sauce
    2 cups fat-free chicken broth
    1/2 medium onion, chopped
    1/2 tsp. ground cumin
    1/2 tsp. chili powder
    1 clove garlic, minced
    Pinch of salt
    12 small corn tortillas
    12 oz. fat-free grated cheese
    1/2 cup fat-free sour cream or yogurt cheese

<u>**Preparation:**</u>

1. Spray skillet with cooking spray. Saute onions and garlic until tender and brown. Add spices and mix, then stir in chicken broth and tomato sauce. Stir and bring to a boil. Reduce heat and simmer for 15 minutes until thickened.

2. Spray a 9 x 13 pan with cooking spray. Fill each corn tortilla with about 1/4 cup cheese and two teaspoons sour cream. Roll up placing seam side down. Spray enchiladas with cooking spray and bake 5 to 7 minutes. Ladle enchilada sauce over and return to the oven for 5 to 7 more minutes.

3. Serve with shredded lettuce and spanish rice.

<u>**Nutritional Analysis per Serving:**</u>

- ♥ 275 calories
- ♥ 27 grams protein
- ♥ 826 mg. sodium

- ♥ 2.4 grams fat
- ♥ 37 grams carbohydrate
- ♥ 4 grams fiber

COLORADO STUFFED PEPPERS

Yield: 4 servings

Ingredients:

3 roma tomatoes, or 2 medium tomatoes, chopped coarsely
1 to 2 cloves garlic, minced
2 green onions, chopped
1 tsp. cumin
1/4 medium red onion, chopped
1/2 sweet red pepper, chopped
1 cup cooked brown rice or bulgur
2 cups cooked black beans or canned black beans
1/4 cup fat-free cheddar cheese
4 bell peppers, seeded and cored

Preparation:

1. Spray pan with cooking spray. Saute tomatoes, onions, garlic, and red pepper in 1 Tbs. water until cooked to desired tenderness.

2. Add brown rice or bulgur, black beans, cumin, and cheese to pan and gently stir until warm and cheese is melted.

3. Meanwhile, cover whole peppers and cook in microwave until tender crisp, about 5 minutes (Cook longer for softer peppers). Fill peppers with bean mixture. Garnish with chopped red pepper, if desired.

Nutritional Analysis per Serving:

- ♥ 217 calories
- ♥ 1 gram fat
- ♥ 16 grams protein
- ♥ 39 grams carbohydrate
- ♥ 121 mg. sodium
- ♥ 7 grams fiber

CREPES

Impress your guests with this versatile french meal that is as easy to make as pancakes!

Yield: 20 crepes

Ingredients:

2 cups white flour
2 Tbs. sugar
1 tsp. vanilla
1 cup + 2 Tbs. water

2 egg whites
1/4 tsp. salt
2 cups skim milk, divided

Preparation:

1. Place flour, egg whites, sugar, salt, 1 cup skim milk and vanilla in bowl. Mix well by hand or with beater. While still mixing, add in 1 cup milk and 1 cup water + 2 Tbs. Beat at medium speed until well mixed.

2. Spray a 10-inch nonstick skillet with cooking spray. Place skillet on stovetop over MEDIUM-HIGH heat. When pan is hot, pour a scant 1/4 cup of batter into pan, turning pan at the same time to cover. (It's all in the wrist!)

3. Cook $1^{1}/_{2}$ minutes until bottom of crepe is golden brown. Use plastic spatula to gently lift up sides of crepe. You can then either turn the crepe with the spatula or flip the crepe up in the air and over. Cook 30 more seconds until other side is brown.

Note: It is important to use a pan that is unscratched to keep crepes from sticking. The first crepe is never perfect and usually goes to the dog! After making a batch of crepes, you will learn which thickness and cooking time you prefer. The batter can be saved for up to a week in the refrigerator. The batter will separate, so when ready to use again, mix with wire whip or electric beater. Cooked crepes can be kept in the refrigerator or freezer by layering between wax paper.

Fillings:

Breakfast / Dessert:

- Fleishman's liquid nonfat margarine or Ultra Fat-Free Promise
- Honey, jam, granulated or powdered sugar, cinnamon sugar
- Fresh or canned fruit of your choice (sliced strawberries, bananas and blueberries work well)
- Canned pie filling
- Liqueur such as Triple Sec, Amaretto, Kahlua
- Fat-free yogurt or sorbet

Lunch / Brunch / Dinner:

- Spring Vegetables with Cream Sauce (page 300)
- Delightful Spinach (page 306)
- Ratatouille (page 309)
- Steamed vegetables with Curry Sauce (page 276)
- Vegetables and prepared lowfat spaghetti sauce
- Flavored black beans and salsa
- Filling from Spinach Stuffed Shells (page 299)
- Tofu filling from Vegetable Lasagna (page 303) + vegetables of your choice

Nutritional Analysis per Serving (4 crepes, no filling):

- ♥ 244 calories
- ♥ 0.7 gram fat
- ♥ 10 grams protein
- ♥ 48 grams carbohydrate
- ♥ 180 mg. sodium

CRUSTLESS QUICHE

Yield: 4 servings

Ingredients:

10 egg whites
1 cup evaporated skim milk
1-10 oz. package spinach, thawed
4 oz. fat-free mozzarella cheese
1 tsp. Italian seasoning
1/3 tsp. salt
1/4 tsp. garlic powder

Preparation:

1. Preheat oven to 350°.
2. Beat egg whites, milk and spices together until frothy. Fold in spinach and cheese.
3. Spray 10-inch pie pan with cooking spray. Pour egg mixture into pan and bake for 45 to 50 minutes.

Variation:, Use 1 cup of any leftover vegetables. Add water chestnuts and low sodium soy sauce for oriental flavor.

Nutritional Analysis per Serving:

- ♥ 170 calories
- ♥ 0.3 gram fat
- ♥ 26 grams protein
- ♥ 15 grams carbohydrate
- ♥ 750 mg. sodium

FAUX FAJITAS

<u>**Yield:**</u> 3 servings

1-8 oz. package Seitan, traditionally seasoned
  (found in refrigerated section of natural foods store)
2 Tbs. water
1 medium onion, cut in half, then sliced
1 medium red pepper, sliced thinly
1 to 2 cloves fresh garlic, minced
1/2 tsp. chili powder
1 tsp. cumin
1/4 tsp. pepper
6 small flour tortillas
Lettuce, tomato, salsa, fat-free cheese, fat-free sour cream, onion

<u>Preparation:</u>

1. Preheat oven to 350°. Heat 2 Tbs. water over MEDIUM heat. Add onion and garlic; cook 3 to 4 minutes. Add spices and red pepper and cook until vegetables are tender, adding more water if necessary. Add drained seitan and cook another 5 minutes.

2. Stack tortillas and sprinkle top one with a few drops of water. Wrap in foil and bake until warm--about 10 minutes.

3. To serve, fill a tortilla with seitan-veggie mixture. Top with shredded lettuce, chopped tomato, onion, salsa, fat-free cheese and fat-free sour cream.

<u>Nutritional Analysis per Serving:</u>

- ♥ 322 calories
- ♥ 27 grams protein
- ♥ 163 mg. sodium
- ♥ 3.7 grams fat
- ♥ 46 grams carbohydrate
- ♥ 3 grams fiber

HAPPY FAMILY DINNER

Yield: 8-1$^1/_2$ cups servings

Vegetables:

4 cups broccoli florets

2 cups sliced mushrooms

1$^1/_2$ cups carrots, sliced

1/2 cup sliced water chestnuts

1 cup whole baby corn, canned

4 cloves fresh garlic, minced

2 cups bok choy, thinly sliced

2 cups snow peas

4 green onions, sliced

1/2 cup fat-free chicken broth

3 tsp. fresh ginger, minced

1 lb. cubed firm tofu (optional)

Sauce:

1$^1/_2$ cups fat-free chicken broth

1 to 2 Tbs. soy sauce

Small amount white pepper

2 to 3 Tbs. dry sherry

3 Tbs. cornstarch or arrowroot

Preparation:

1. Combine sauce ingredients in a separate bowl and set aside.

2. Brown optional tofu in non-stick pan for 5 to 10 minutes.

3. In a wok or large saucepan, place about 1/2 cup broth. Heat until it boils; add garlic, ginger and green onions. Cook 2 minutes. Then add broccoli, and carrots. Cook and stir for about 10 minutes. Add mushrooms, bok choy and snow peas. Cook and stir for 3 to 5 minutes. Add water chestnuts and cook a few more minutes.

4. Add sauce mixture to pan. Bring to a boil, stirring constantly. After mixture boils and thickens, stir in baby corn, add optional tofu.

5. Serving Suggestion: Serve over brown rice or noodles.

Nutritional Analysis per Serving:

- ♥ 117 calories
- ♥ 6.2 grams protein
- ♥ 578 mg. sodium
- ♥ 0.9 gram fat
- ♥ 24 grams carbohydrate
- ♥ 5.7 grams fiber

HOPPIN' JOHN

<u>Yield:</u> 4-1³/₄ cups servings

<u>Ingredients:</u>

   3 cups cooked bulgur or brown rice
   1-16 oz. can kidney beans
   1-16 oz. can black eyed peas
   1-10 oz. package frozen sliced okra, thawed (optional)
   1 medium onion, chopped
   1 bay leaf
   1 tsp. dried thyme
   1/2 tsp. pepper

<u>Preparation:</u>

1. Spray pan with cooking spray. Add onion, and spices. Add 1 to 2 Tbs. of water and cook until onion is tender. (If using okra, add here and cook 5 minutes until warm.) Add beans with their liquid. Simmer 10 minutes or more.

2. Stir in bulgur. Cook until warmed through.

<u>Nutritional Analysis per Serving:</u>

- ♥ 326 calories
- ♥ 1.5 grams fat
- ♥ 17 grams protein
- ♥ 65 grams carbohydrate
- ♥ 718 mg. sodium
- ♥ 11 grams fiber

MILLET BURGERS

Patty Magliato introduced us to millet with this recipe. It's even a favorite with kids!

Yield: 8 small burgers; 4 servings

Ingredients:

1 cup millet, uncooked
1/8 tsp. cayenne pepper, or other spice
Cooking spray
2 cups water
1 tsp. salt (optional)
1 cup grated carrot
1/2 cup onion, minced
1/2 cup fresh parsley, minced
1/2 to 3/4 cup whole wheat flour

Preparation:

1. Spray skillet with cooking spray. Heat over MEDIUM heat briefly; add millet and spice. Roast until fragrant, 2 to 3 minutes.

2. Add 2 cups water and salt; bring to a boil. Simmer until water is absorbed, 35 to 40 minutes.

3. Preheat oven to 375°. Pour millet into a bowl and let cool. Add last 4 ingredients and mix with a spoon or hands. Form into 8 patties.

4. Bake 10 minutes on each side.

5. Serve on a bun with all the trimmings.

Nutritional Analysis per Serving:

- 219 calories
- 7 grams protein
- 17 mg. sodium
- 1.8 grams fat
- 45 grams carbohydrate
- 9 grams fiber

MOCK EGG FOO YUNG

__Yield__: 8-2 oz. patties

Ingredients:

16 oz. lowfat firm tofu crumbled
2 egg whites
6 Tbs. cornmeal or seasoned bread crumbs
1 Tbs. low-salt soy sauce
3/4 tsp. fresh ginger, finely grated
4 green onions, finely chopped
2 large cloves garlic, finely minced
1/4 tsp. sesame oil
1 medium sized carrot, finely grated
1/2 cup mung bean sprouts, cut in half
1 Tbs. sesame seeds

Preparation:

1. Squeeze out extra water from tofu. Mix all ingredients except last 3. Fold in last ingredients until just blended. Form into 8 small patties.

2. Spray pan with cooking spray. Cook patties on both sides until lightly browned.

3. Serve with sweet and sour sauce, teriyaki sauce, or sauce from Happy Family Dinner.

Nutritional Analysis per Serving:

- ♥ 135 calories
- ♥ 3.3 grams fat
- ♥ 12 grams protein
- ♥ 15 grams carbohydrate
- ♥ 269 mg. sodium

OAT NUT BURGERS

Yield: 6 burgers

Ingredients:

2/3 cup rolled oats (not instant)
1/3 cup chopped cashews
1 onion, chopped
3 stalks celery, chopped
2 carrots grated (or 1 carrot and 1/3 zucchini, grated)
1/4 cup each whole wheat flour and water
1 tsp. low sodium soy sauce (optional)
Salt and pepper to taste

Preparation:

1. Mix all ingredients. Season to taste with soy sauce or salt and pepper.
2. Shape into 6 burgers. Cook in pan sprayed with cooking spray--about 10 minutes on each side, or broil in oven.
3. Serve on a bun with all the trimmings.

Nutritional Analysis per Serving:

- ♥ 117 calories
- ♥ 4.4 grams fat
- ♥ 4 grams protein
- ♥ 15 grams carbohydrate
- ♥ 24 mg. sodium
- ♥ 3 grams fiber

PASTA E FAGIOL

<u>Yield:</u> 6 servings

Ingredients:

32 oz. prepared lowfat pasta sauce
1-8 oz. can "pasta ready" Italian style tomatoes
2-15 oz. cans water packed red kidney beans, drain and rinsed
1 tsp. Italian seasoning
1 to 2 cloves garlic, minced
1 pound uncooked egg-free whole wheat or spinach pasta

Preparation:

1. Preheat oven to 350°. Place all the ingredients except the pasta in a large bowl. Stir until blended. Cook the pasta separately according to directions, and drain.

2. Combine the sauce with the pasta in a 3-quart casserole dish and bake for 20 minutes.

Nutritional Analysis per Serving:

- ♥ 437 calories
- ♥ 3.3 grams fat
- ♥ 20 grams protein
- ♥ 86 grams carbohydrate
- ♥ 13 grams fiber

PASTA WITH QUICK ALFREDO SAUCE

Yield: 4-2 cups servings

Ingredients:

1$^1/_2$ cups fat-free cottage cheese
1/2 cup skim milk
1/2 tsp. garlic powder or 2 cloves fresh garlic, pressed
1 package Butter Buds
2 Tbs. freshly grated parmesan cheese
2 dashes nutmeg
1-10 oz. package frozen peas, thawed
6 cups cooked pasta

Preparation:

1. Puree all ingredients except peas and pasta in food processor or blender.

2. Pour into microwave safe dish and cook on MEDIUM-HIGH for 2 minutes. Or cook over stove, LOW-MEDIUM heat until warm.

3. Toss pasta with peas. Pour sauce over pasta.

Nutritional Analysis per Serving:

- ♥ 421 calories
- ♥ 2.6 grams fat
- ♥ 26 grams protein
- ♥ 72 grams carbohydrate
- ♥ 443 mg. sodium
- ♥ 5 grams fiber

SLOPPY JOES

Recipe from THE SIMPLE SOYBEAN AND YOUR HEALTH by Mark Messina and Virginia Messina. © 1994. Published by Avery Publishing Group, Inc., Garden City Park, New York. Reprinted with permission.

Yield: 4 servings

Ingredients:

> 1 cup TVP (Textured Vegetable Protein)
> (found in bulk at large natural food stores)
> 1 cup boiling water
> 1-16 oz. can sloppy joe sauce
> 4 whole wheat hamburger buns

Preparation:

1. To rehydrate the TVP, place the TVP in a medium saucepan and pour boiling water over it.
2. Add the sloppy joe sauce to the TVP; cook over LOW heat until heated thoroughly.
3. To serve, pour the TVP mixture over the hamburger rolls.

Nutritional Analysis per Serving:

- ♥ 198 calories
- ♥ 2 grams fat
- ♥ 15 grams protein
- ♥ 32 grams carbohydrate
- ♥ 804 mg. sodium

SPINACH STUFFED SHELLS

Yield: 4 servings

Ingredients:

1/2 lb. large pasta shells, cooked until slightly firm
1-10 oz. package frozen spinach, cooked and drained
1 cup fat-free cottage cheese
1/2 cup grated fat-free mozzarella type cheese
2 Tbs. freshly grated parmesan cheese
2 cloves garlic, minced
$1^{1}/_{2}$ tsp. Italian seasoning
1/2 tsp. pepper
2 cups lowfat spaghetti sauce

Preparation:

1. Mix spinach, cheeses and spices until well blended.
2. Stuff each shell with spinach mixture and top with sauce.
3. Bake or microwave until hot.

Nutritional Analysis per Serving:

- ♥ 360 calories
- ♥ 3 grams fat
- ♥ 28 grams protein
- ♥ 55 grams carbohydrate
- ♥ 967 mg. sodium
- ♥ 4 grams fiber

SPRING VEGETABLES IN CREAM SAUCE

<u>Yield:</u> 4-1 cup servings

<u>Sauce:</u>

1$^1/_2$ cups fat-free chicken broth	1 cup skim milk
1 package Butter Buds	3 Tbs. cornstarch
1/2 tsp. tarragon	1/4 tsp. each dill and basil
1/2 tsp. onion powder	1/2 tsp. garlic salt
1 tsp. lemon pepper	1 tsp. lemon juice

<u>Vegetables:</u>

1-1 lb. package Green Giant California Style Vegetables
(has cauliflower, carrots, asparagus) or other vegetable mixture
1-7 or 14 oz. can artichoke hearts, quartered
1/2 red bell pepper, sliced thinly

<u>Preparation:</u>

1. Put chicken broth, milk, cornstarch and butter buds in blender. Blend on high until mixed well. Pour into large saucepan. Add rest of sauce ingredients. Cook over MEDIUM heat, stirring often until thick.

2. Meanwhile, steam vegetables or cook in microwave. Add to thickened sauce.

<u>Serving Suggestions:</u>

Serve over rice, bulgur, or angel hair pasta. Or roll up in a crepe or flour tortilla.

<u>Nutritional Analysis per Serving:</u>

- ♥ 103 calories
- ♥ 5.5 grams protein
- ♥ 550 mg. sodium
- ♥ 0.4 gram fat
- ♥ 22 grams carbohydrate
- ♥ 4 grams fiber

STUFFED EGGPLANT CREOLE

Yield: 4 servings

Ingredients:

2 small eggplants (1 lb. each)
1 lb. firm tofu, cubed
1 clove garlic, crushed
1 14 oz. can tomatoes, undrained
1/4 tsp. thyme
1 cup fat-free sour cream or non-fat yogurt
1/4 cup each: finely chopped onion, green pepper, celery
1 cup dry bread crumbs, plain or Italian
Tabasco or cayenne (optional)

Preparation:

1. Preheat oven to 375°. Wash eggplant, cut in half lengthwise. Place in a large pan. Cover with water. Bring to a boil and cover. Simmer 15 minutes. Drain and cool.

2. Scoop out pulp from eggplant, taking care to leave 1/4 inch of the shell intact.

3. Spray a nonstick skillet with cooking spray. Add vegetables and cook until tender crisp. Add tofu and cook until warm.

4. Stir in tomatoes, salt, thyme, and tabasco if desired. Add half of the bread crumbs. Stir in eggplant and sour cream.

5. Stuff mixture back into 4 eggplant shells. Top with remaining bread crumbs. Place in baking dish and bake for 30 minutes.

Nutritional Analysis per Serving:

- ♥ 290 calories
- ♥ 3.5 grams fat
- ♥ 49 grams carbohydrate
- ♥ 5 grams fiber

TOFU LOAF

This recipe is from Norma Robinson. The pecans give it an interesting texture and flavor.

Yield: 8 slices

Ingredients:

16 oz. lowfat firm tofu
1/4 cup chopped pecans
1/2 cup canned tomatoes, chopped
2 egg whites
1/4 cup skim milk
1/2 cup dry bread crumbs, plain or seasoned
1/2 tsp. salt
1/2 tsp. each onion and garlic powder
1 tsp. thyme, cumin, oregano or Italian seasoning
Optional seasonings: chopped parsley, green onion, finely chopped celery or onion.

Preparation:

1. Preheat oven to 350°. Squeeze out excess liquid from tofu and crumble. With a spoon, mix with rest of ingredients until well blended. Pour into loaf pan that has been sprayed with cooking spray. Bake 50 to 60 minutes.

2. Serve like meat loaf with ketchup, salsa, pasta sauce or on a bun like a burger. Leftovers are great as sandwiches.

Nutritional Analysis per Serving:

- 86 calories
- 8 grams protein
- 5 grams carbohydrate
- 4.2 grams fat
- 346 mg. sodium

VEGETABLE LASAGNA

This recipe was inspired by Patty Magliato. It uses uncooked noodles to save time.

Yield: 9 servings

Marinara Sauce:

2-28 oz. cans Progresso Italian Style Tomatoes with basil
1-28 oz. can no added salt tomato sauce
3 to 4 large cloves garlic, minced
2 tsp. basil
2 tsp. Italian seasoning
Pinch sugar
Salt and pepper to taste

Lasagna:

2 pounds firm lowfat tofu
1/4 cup lemon juice
1 tsp. fennel seeds
1 Tbs. honey
2 to 3 cloves garlic, minced
1 tsp. each dried oregano and basil
1-8 oz. package regular or whole wheat lasagna noodles
1-10 oz. package frozen broccoli, thawed
1 medium zucchini, sliced thinly
2 carrots, grated
4 oz. fresh mushrooms, thinly sliced

Preparation:

1. To make sauce, pour both cans of tomatoes in food processor or blender. Process until smooth. Pour into saucepan and add tomato sauce and spices. Simmer 15 to 20 minutes.

2. While sauce is cooking, squeeze extra liquid from tofu. Put in bowl of food processor; add lemon juice, honey and spice. Process until well mixed. In microwave safe dish, gently mix vegetables together. Cover and cook in microwave 6 to 8 minutes, until tender. Pour into colander to drain excess liquid.

3. Preheat oven to 375°. To assemble, spray 9 x 13 inch pan with cooking spray. Do not cook noodles. Spread 1 cup of the sauce in the bottom of the pan. Lay down 3 noodles side-by-side. Spread 1 cup of sauce. Spread 1/2 of tofu and 1/2 of vegetable mixture. Add 1 cup of sauce. Add 3 noodles and press down. Spread 1 cup of sauce over noodles, then spoon the remaining tofu and vegetables. Top with 1 cup of sauce. Lay down last of noodles and press down. Cover with remaining sauce, making sure that all noodles are covered.

Nutritional Analysis per Serving:

- ♥ 236 calories
- ♥ 2.2 grams fat
- ♥ 15 grams protein
- ♥ 41 grams carbohydrate
- ♥ 413 mg. sodium
- ♥ 5 grams fiber

BULGUR AND VEGGIE MIX

Yield: 5-1 cup servings

Ingredients:

1 cup dry bulgur
2$^1/_2$ cups chopped broccoli, or other vegetable in season
2 cups water
1/4 tsp. salt
1/2 tsp. thyme

Preparation:

1. Bring water to boil. Add salt. Add broccoli. Simmer 5 minutes.
2. Place bulgur in heat-proof serving bowl. Pour water and broccoli over bulgur.
3. Cover and let sit until most of the water is absorbed.
4. Pour off excess water and fluff with a fork.

Variation:

Any vegetable, or combination, fresh or frozen, can be used in place of the broccoli. California style vegetable mix (frozen) also works well.

Nutritional Analysis per Serving:

- ♥ 103 calories
- ♥ 0.5 gram fat
- ♥ 5.6 grams protein
- ♥ 22 grams carbohydrate
- ♥ 148 mg. sodium
- ♥ 6 grams fiber

DELIGHTFUL SPINACH

<u>Yield:</u> 4-1 cup servings

<u>Ingredients:</u>

2-10 oz. package frozen chopped spinach, thawed or cooked, or 2 lb.
   fresh spinach or other green, cooked
8 oz. fat-free cream cheese
1 tsp. mixed herbs (Italian seasoning, herbs de Provence, etc.)
Pepper, to taste
2 drops tabasco sauce (optional)

<u>Preparation:</u>

1. In a nonstick saucepan, cook cream cheese and spices together until
   melted. Squeeze out excess water from spinach. Add to cream cheese.
2. Cook until warmed through.

<u>Serving Suggestion:</u>

Serve over rice, on pizza or stuffed in a crepe or tortilla.

<u>Nutritional Analysis per Serving:</u>

- ♥ 76 calories
- ♥ 0.2 gram fat
- ♥ 11 grams protein
- ♥ 9 grams carbohydrate
- ♥ 466 mg. sodium

GREEK PILAF

Yield: 7-2/3 cup servings

Ingredients:

$1^1/_2$ cups long grain brown rice
$1^1/_2$ cups minced onion
1/2 tsp. salt
1 tsp. black pepper
2 Tbs. lemon juice
1 Tbs. dried mint

$2^1/_2$ cups water
1 small stalk celery, minced
1/2 cup sunflower seeds or pine nuts
4 medium cloves garlic, minced
1/4 cup freshly minced parsley

Preparation:

1. Place the rice and water in a saucepan. Bring to a boil, cover, and simmer until tender (40 to 45 minutes).
2. Heat 2 Tbs. of water in a small skillet. Add onion, celery, and salt, and saute until tender, adding more water as necessary (5 to 8 minutes). Add sunflower seeds or pine nuts, black pepper, and garlic. Saute for 5 minutes.
3. Stir the sauteed mixture into the cooked rice along with the lemon juice and herbs. Mix well.

Time Saver:

Use bulgur wheat instead, cook 10 minutes. Or use instant brown rice.

Nutritional Analysis per Serving:

- ♥ 194 calories
- ♥ 3.7 grams fat
- ♥ 5 grams protein
- ♥ 36 grams carbohydrate
- ♥ 162 mg. sodium
- ♥ 3 grams fiber

OVEN FRIED POTATOES

Yield: 4-6 servings

Ingredients:

6 medium potatoes, (peeled or unpeeled) and sliced thinly
Cooking spray
Your choice of seasonings: garlic powder, Italian seasoning, cajun spice mix, chili powder and cumin, seasoned salt, Mrs. Dash

Preparation:

1. Preheat oven to 350°. Spray cookie sheet with cooking spray.

2. Place potatoes on cookie sheet, spray lightly with cooking spray and sprinkle with desired spices. Bake for about 20 minutes or to desired brownness, turning once.

3. For extra crisp potatoes, slice paper thin. For "home fries" slice thicker or in wedges.

Nutritional Analysis per Serving:

- ♥ 217 calories
- ♥ 0.2 gram fat
- ♥ 4.6 grams protein
- ♥ 50 grams carbohydrate
- ♥ 11 mg. sodium
- ♥ 5 grams fiber

RATATOUILLE

Yield: 8-1 cup servings

Ingredients:

4 cloves garlic, crushed
8 tomatoes, quartered
3 zucchini, sliced
1 eggplant, peeled and cut into 1 inch cubes
1 cup sliced mushrooms
1 tsp. oregano
1 tsp. basil
Salt and pepper to taste

Preparation:

1. Spray nonstick pan with cooking spray. Brown eggplant, adding 1 tablespoon of water at a time as needed. Cook until tender. Add remaining ingredients.

2. Cook over MEDIUM heat until vegetables are tender, stirring frequently.

3. Reduce heat, cover and simmer 10 to 15 minutes. Remove cover and continue cooking until most of the liquid has evaporated.

Nutrient Analysis per Serving:

♥ 58 calories

♥ 1 gram Fat

♥ 2 grams protein

♥ 12 grams carbohydrates

♥ 15 mg. sodium

♥ 4 grams fiber

BANANAS FOSTER

Yield: 6 servings

Ingredients:

4 bananas
1 Tbs. lemon juice
1 package butter buds
3 Tbs. water
2 Tbs. orange juice
2/3 cup brown sugar
3 to 4 Tbs. dark rum
1 tsp. cinnamon

Preparation:

1. Mix butter buds, orange juice and water in nonstick skillet. Add brown sugar and cook until thick and bubbly, stirring often. Add bananas, spooning sauce over until warm. Add rum and flame. Sprinkle cinnamon over flame; this will create sparks which is mostly for show.

2. Serve over nonfat vanilla frozen yogurt.

Nutritional Analysis per Serving: (bananas and sauce only)

- ♥ 191 calories
- ♥ 0.4 gram fat
- ♥ 1 gram protein
- ♥ 45 grams carbohydrate
- ♥ 9 mg. sodium

CARAMEL DIP

This is Cindy McKee's recipe for a dip you won't believe is fat-free! Try with sliced apples or other fresh fruit or on graham crackers.

Yield: 8-2 Tbs. servings

Ingredients:

    8 oz. fat-free cream cheese
    1/3 cup brown sugar, packed
    1 tsp. Watkin's Caramel Flavor
    1 tsp. Vanilla

Preparation:

1. Mix all ingredients with mixer. Chill and serve.

Nutrient Analysis per Serving:

- ♥ 57 Calories
- ♥ 0 Fat
- ♥ 4 g. protein
- ♥ 11 grams carbohydrate
- ♥ 192 mg. sodium

Note: Watkins Caramel Flavor can be ordered by calling 1-800-247-5907, Director #47233.

CHOCOLATE ALMOND DREAM

Yield: 5-3/4 cup servings

Ingredients:

8 oz. fat free cream cheese
1 cup powdered sugar
1/2 cup Cool Whip Lite
3/4 tsp. almond extract
1 small package instant chocolate pudding mix
$1^3/_4$ cups skim milk
1/4 cup crushed graham crackers, grapenuts or fat-free granola

Preparation:

1. In small bowl beat cream cheese until smooth. Add powdered sugar and almond extract and mix well. Fold in cool whip.

2. In another small bowl, mix milk and pudding mix according to package directions.

3. In wine or dessert glasses, put small amount of pudding, a larger layer of cream cheese mixture and another layer of chocolate pudding. Top with graham cracker crumbs or other crunchy topping.

4. Refrigerate at least 1/2 hour before serving.

Nutritional Analysis per Serving:

- ♥ 275 calories
- ♥ 3.2 grams fat
- ♥ 9 grams protein
- ♥ 54 grams carbohydrate
- ♥ 722 mg. sodium

EASY PEACH COBBLER

Yield: 6 servings

Ingredients:

1 cup flour
2/3 cup sugar
$1^1/_2$ tsp. baking powder
1/2 tsp. salt
1-21 oz. can lite Peach pie filling
1 tsp. almond flavoring
3/4 cup canned evaporated skim milk
1 package butter buds (not diluted)

Preparation:

1. Preheat oven to 350°. Spray 2 quart casserole dish with cooking spray.
2. Mix together flour, sugar, baking powder, salt, butter buds, almond flavoring and milk. Pour into casserole.
3. Spoon pie filling on top.
4. Bake at 350° for 35 to 40 minutes or until golden brown.

Serving Suggestion:

Serve warm with non-fat frozen yogurt

Variation:

Blueberry or apple pie filling also work well. If you like alot more fruit than crust, use 2 cans of pie filling and put into dish first, topped with batter.

Nutritional Analysis per Serving:

- 275 Calories
- 4.6 grams protein
- 0.4 gram fat
- 64 grams carbohydrate

TIRAMISU

This light dessert is great for company. If you're not keen on coffee, try the fruit variation.

Yield: 8 servings

Ingredients:

8 oz. fat-free cream cheese
2/3 cup powdered sugar
1/2 cup fat-free sour cream
1/3 cup sugar
3 Tbs. water
2 egg whites
3/4 cup hot water
$1^1/_2$ Tbs. sugar
1 Tbs. + 1 tsp. instant coffee granules
1/4 cup Kahlua or other coffee liqueur
15 lady fingers
3 Tbs. unsweetened cocoa.

Preparation

1. Mix cheese, sour cream and powdered sugar in a bowl at high speed with electric mixer.

2. In the top of a double boiler over simmering water, combine next 3 ingredients. Beat at high speed until stiff peaks form. Gently fold in 1/4 of egg white mixture into cream mixture. Gradually fold in rest of egg white mixture.

3. Combine next 4 ingredients in small bowl. Arrange 15 lady finger halves, cut side up in 8 x 8 pan. (size of ladyfingers may vary, so you may need more or less to cover pan.) Drizzle 1/2 of coffee mixture over ladyfinger halves. Spread half of cream cheese mixture over ladyfingers. Repeat procedure with remaining ladyfingers and cream cheese mixture.

4. Sprinkle cocoa over top, using sifter or strainer. Place one toothpick in each corner and cover with plastic wrap. Chill or freeze 2 hours before serving.

Nutritional Analysis per Serving:

- ♥ 196 calories
- ♥ 0.8 gram fat
- ♥ 7 grams protein
- ♥ 37 grams carbohydrate
- ♥ 317 mg. sodium

Fruit Variation:

Instead of hot water, sugar and instant coffee, use raspberry juice or other fruit juice. Instead of kahlua, use fruit flavored liquor such as kirsch or Triple Sec. Instead of sour cream, use strawberry or raspberry nonfat yogurt. On top of ladyfingers that have been drizzled with juice-liqueur mixture, lay sliced strawberries or raspberries. Omit cocoa and garnish top with sliced fruit.

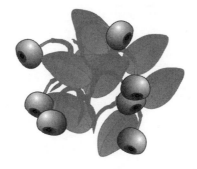

VERY BERRY SHAKE

<u>**Yield:**</u> 2-1 cup servings

<u>**Ingredients:**</u>

    1 cup frozen sweetened berries, any combination
        (blueberry and strawberry is good)
    1 cup nonfat vanilla yogurt

<u>**Preparation:**</u>

1. Blend all and serve.

<u>**Variation:**</u>

You can also use any combination of any fruit, fresh or frozen. If using fresh, freeze first. Cut the sugar by using sugar-free yogurt and unsweetened berries. Good combinations of fruit include:

Banana and strawberry

Pineapple and coconut flavoring

Apple and apple pie spice

Chocolate syrup and frozen nonfat yogurt

<u>**Nutritional Analysis per Serving:**</u>

- ♥ 189 calories
- ♥ 0.2 gram fat
- ♥ 6 grams protein
- ♥ 44 grams carbohydrate
- ♥ 71 mg. sodium

CHAPTER 15

CHOICES

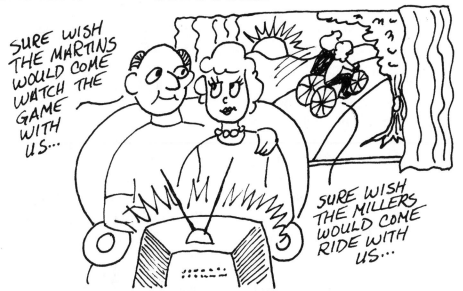

THE CHOICE IS YOURS—
"ARMCHAIR ATHLETE" OR "EVERYDAY ATHLETE"

Alice: "Would you tell me, please, which way I ought to go from here?"

Cat: "That depends a good deal on where you want to get."

Alice: "I don't much care..."

Cat: "Then it doesn't matter which way to go."

Alice: "So long as I get somewhere."

Cat: "Oh, you are sure to do that if you only walk long enough."

Alice in Wonderland by Lewis Carroll

Your life is filled with choices. Your future, to a large degree, will be affected by the choices you make today.

Learn to make choices that are best for your overall happiness and well-being. Learn from your mistakes. Keep the big picture in mind.

Many people are miserable today because of bad choices: in business, in love, in health. The natural order is so resilient, however, that they often get a second chance. As my friend Paul Smith always says, "opportunity only knocks three or four times!"

Our bodies are built for survival. As human beings we can and should expect more than survival. Good health and happiness can be achieved. You don't have to be caught, trapped in the hamster's cage. Open up to new ideas. Enjoy life to the fullest!

At the Preventive Health Institute, we have helped people like you make some of these hard choices.

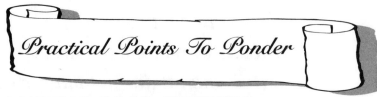

Practical Points To Ponder

MAKING GOOD CHOICES

- ♥ Will I be happy, or will I settle for content?
- ♥ Is my glass half full or half empty? Do I have an upbeat attitude?
- ♥ Will I be fit or fat?

- ♥ Will practice of self awareness and control govern my actions, or will stress make me explode?
- ♥ Will I live as a human being, with all the blemishes, or always expect perfection?
- ♥ Should I eat to live, or continue to live to eat?
- ♥ Should I use my body, and improve in health, or lose it, and get even sicker?
- ♥ Am I happy with myself, with who I really am? If not, what am I willing to change?
- ♥ Should I continue to put up with abuse from my spouse and family?
- ♥ Should I cut back and enjoy life, or continue to "kill myself" for my work or my boss?

Stress reduction and group support help people like you work through and resolve these dilemmas. Practice making the right choices for you!

<u>Take this test:</u>

At the end of your natural life, after the funeral, at the grave, what will you want on your tombstone?

- ♥ "I didn't work hard enough."
- ♥ "I didn't gather enough toys."
- ♥ "I didn't get to eat everything I wanted."
- ♥ "I loved my spouse, my family, my community."
- ♥ "I died having experienced great happiness."
- ♥ "I contributed all I possibly could during my short life, and I hope others will say it was enough."

You often read when others develop a terminal illness, they feel a heightened sense of life. They develop the ability to live life to the fullest, savoring all that comes in their path. No event seems too small or insignificant to enjoy!

Your time is short. Why not focus on what is important, and with all your energy, work toward that personal goal. Don't be diverted, just do it!

After you determine what is important, I hope this book helps make you "feel like doing it." There are many ways to live life. Since we only go around once, why not feel good about it? Only you can answer that question.

POSTSCRIPT

We are most interested in what you choose and how you come to "feel like doing it." Please write us with your comments, and share your success with others:

Frank Barry, MD
C/O Preventive Health Institute
2130 Hollowbrook
Colorado Springs, Colorado 80918

or fax:

(719) 590-7037

REFERENCES

1. Ornstein R, Sobel D. *Healthy Pleasures*. New York: Addison-Wesley; 1989.

2. Jones PH, Gotto AM Jr. Prevention of Coronary Heart Disease in 1994... *Heart Dis Stroke*. 1994; 3(6):290-6.

3. Ornish DM. The Lifestyle Heart Trial. *Lancet*. 1990; 336:129-133.

4. Watts GF et al. Effects on coronary artery disease... in the St. Thomas atherosclerosis regression study. *Lancet*. 1992; 339:563-569.

5. The Coronary Drug Project Research Group. Clofibrate and niacin in coronary heart disease. *JAMA*. 1975; 231:360-381.

6. The Pravastatin Multinational Study Group for Cardiac Risk Patients. Effects of pravastatin... *Am J Cardiol*. 1993; 72(14):1031-1037.

7. Brown G. Regression of coronary artery disease... *N Engl J Med*. 1990; 323(19):1289-1298.

8. Blankenhorn DH et al. Beneficial effects of combined colestipol-niacin therapy... *JAMA*. 1987; 257:3233-3240.

9. Pedersen T. Scandinavian simmstatin study group. The Scandinavian simmstatin survival study. *Lancet*. 1994; 344:(45)1383-1389.

10. Kannel WB, Abbott RD. Incidence and prognosis of unrecognized myocardial infarction: an update on the framingham study. *N Engl J Med*. 1984; 311(18):1144.

11. Hamm CW. A randomized study of coronary angioplasty compared with bypass surgery... *N Engl J Med*. 1994; 331:(16)1037-1043.

12. Ridolphi RL. The relationship between coronary artery lesions and myocardial infarcts: ulceration of atherosclerotic plaques precipitating coronary thrombosis. *Am Heart J*. 1977; 93(4):468-486.

13. Arca M et al. Hypercholesterolemia in Postmenopausal Women. *JAMA*. 1994; 271(6):453-59.

14. SHEP Cooperative Research Group. Prevention of stroke by antihypertensive drug treatment. *JAMA*. 1991; 265(24):3255-64.

15. Unpublished study, American Heart Association Meeting, University of Washington at the AHA, 1995.

16. Hunninghake DB et al. The efficacy of intensive dietary therapy... *N Engl J Med*. 1993; 328(17):1213-19.

17. Giovanucci E et al. A Prospective study of dietary fat and risk of prostate cancer. *J Natl Cancer Inst*. 1993; 85(19):1571-9.

18. Howe GR et al. Dietary factors and risk of breast cancer... *J Natl Cancer Inst*. 1990; 82(7):561-69.

19. Gould KL et al. Short term cholesterol lowering... *Circulation*. 1994; 89(4):1530-38.

20. Fischer L. "The Low Cholesterol Gourmet" quoted in the *Colorado Springs Gazette Telegraph*. Sept. 28, 1994; p: 2 Lifestyle section.

21. Zemel MB. Calcium utilization: effect of varying level and source of dietary protein. *Am J Clin Nutr*. 1988; 48:880-883.

22. Campbell Wetal. Increased protein requirements in elderly people... *Am J Clin Nutr*. 1994; 60:50-9.

23. Morris DL et al. Serum carotenoids and coronary heart disease. *JAMA*. 1994; 272(18)1439-41.

24. Zemel MB. Calcium utilization... *Am J Clin Nutr*. 1988; 48: 880-883.

25. Kerstetter JE, Allen LH. Dietary Protein increases urinary calcium. *J Nutr*. 1990; 120:134-136.

26. Frahm A. *A Cancer Battle Plan*. Colorado Springs, CO; Pinon Press; 1992.

27. Verrillo A et al. Soybean protein diets in the management of Type II hyperlipoproteinemia. *Atherosclerosis*. 1985; 54:321-331.

28. Bresslau NA. Relationship of animal protein-rich diet to kidney stone formation and calcium metabolism. *J Clin Endocrinol Metab*. 1988; 66:140-146.

29. Havala S, Clifford M. *Simple, Lowfat and Vegetarian; Unbelievably Easy Ways to Reduce the Fat in Your Meals*. Baltimore; MD: Vegetarian Resource Group; 1994.

30. Green LA, Ruffin MT. A closer examination of sex bias... *J Fam Pract*. 1994; 39:(4)331-6.

31. Shaw LJ et al. Gender differences in the noninvasive evaluation of... *Ann Int Med*. 1994; 120:(7)559-66.

32. Stampfer MJ et al. A prospective study of postmenopausal estrogen therapy. *N Engl J Med*. 1985; 313;1044-9.

33. Bush TL et al. Cardiovascular mortality and noncontraceptive use of estrogen in women. *Circulation*. 1987; 75(6):1102-1109.

34. Riggs BL, Seeman E. Effect of the fluoride--calcium regimen on vertebral fracture in postmenopausal osteoporosis. *NEJM*. 1982; 306(8):446-450.

35. National Institute of Health Consensus Conference, Optimal Calcium Intake. *JAMA*. 1994; 272(24):1942.

36. Cancer Statistics. *CA Cancer Clinical Journal* 1994; 44:7-26.

37. Gambrell, RD.*The Menopause*. London: Blackwell Scientific Publications Ltd.; 1988: 247.

38. Dupont WD, Page DL. Menopausal estrogen replacement therapy and breast cancer. *Arch Intern Med*. 1991; 151:(1)67.

39. Moliterno DJ et al. Coronary vasoconstriction... *N Engl J Med* 1994; 330(7):454-9.

40. Kawachi I et al. Symptoms of anxiety and risk of coronary heart disease. *Circulation*. 1994; 90(5):2225-29.

41. Carney RM et al. Major depressive disorder predicts cardiac events in patients with coronary artery disease. *Psychosom Med*. 1988; 50(6):627.

42. Prochaska JO. The transtheoretical model. *Am Psychol*. 1992; 47:1102-1114.

43. Kelly G. Antihypertensive effects of aerobic exercise. *Am J Hypertens.* 1994; 7:115-119.

44. Blair SN et al. Physical fitness and all cause mortality. *JAMA* 1989; 262(17):2395-2401.

45. Glynn TJ. The Fagerstrom Tolerance Test in *How to Help Your Patients Stop Smoking.* Washington D.C.: National Institute of Health; 1990. NIH publication 90-3064.

46. Selhub J et al. Vitamin status as primary determinants of homocysteinemia in an elderly population. *JAMA.* 1993; 270(22):2693-98.

47. Stampfer MJ et al. Vitamin E consumption and the risk of coronary artery disease in women. *N Engl J Med* 1993; 328(20):1444-49.

48. Selhub J et al. Association between plasma homocysteine concentrations and extracranial carotid artery stenosis. *N Engl J Med.* 1995; 332(5):286-291.

49. Press R et al. The role of chromium picolinate on serum cholesterol and apolipoprotein factions in human subjects. *West J Med* 1990; 152:41-45.

50. Reiser S et al. Indices of copper status in humans... *Am J Clin Nutr.* 1985; 42(2):242-251.

51. Kessler D. Therapeutic class wars-drug promotion in a competitive marketplace. *N Engl Journ Med.* 1994; 331(20):1350-1353.

52. Alavanja MC et al. Saturated fat intake and lung cancer risk... *J Natl Cancer Inst.* 1993; 85(23):1906-1916.

53. Howe GR et al. Dietary factors and risk of breast cancer... *J Natl Cancer Inst.* 1990; 82(7):561-69.

54. Giovannucci E et al. A prospective study of dietary fat and risk of prostate cancer. *J Natl Cancer Inst.* 1993; 85(19):1571-79.

55. Trock B et al. Dietary Fiber, vegetables, and colon cancer... *J Natl Cancer Inst.* 1990; 82(8):650-61.

SUGGESTED READINGS

FOREWORD

- ♥ The works of Nathan Pritiken.
- ♥ The many books by Kenneth Cooper, MD.
- ♥ The works of John McDougall, MD and Mary McDougall.
- ♥ Frahm A. *A Cancer Battle Plan.* Colorado Springs, CO: Pinon Press; 1992.
- ♥ Ornish D. *Reversing Heart Disease.* New York. Ballantine; 1990.

CHAPTER 1--21ST CENTURY MEDICINE

- ♥ Ornstein D, Sobel R. *Healthy Pleasures.* New York: Addison-Wesley, 1989.
- ♥ Jones PH, Gotto AM Jr. Prevention of Coronary Heart Disease in 1994... *Heart Dis Stroke.* 1994; 3(6):290-6.

CHAPTER 2--THE PROBLEM WITH HEART DISEASE

- ♥ Kessler D. Therapeutic class wars-drug promotion in a competitive marketplace. *N Engl J Med.* 1994; 331(20):1350-1353.
- ♥ Arca M et al. Hypercholesterolemia in Postmenopausal Women. *JAMA.* 1994; 271(6):453-59.
- ♥ Pekkanen J et al. Ten year mortality... *N Engl J Med.* 1990; 322(24):1700-1707.
- ♥ Hunninghake DB et al. The efficacy of intensive dietary therapy... *N Engl J Med.* 1993; 328(17):1213-19.
- ♥ Bachinsky WB. Angioplasty in Multivessel Coronary Artery Disease. *Hosp Pract Off Ed.* 1994; 29(12):27-33.
- ♥ SHEP Cooperative Research Group. Prevention of stroke by antihypertensive drug treatment. *JAMA.* 1991; 265(24):3255-64.
- ♥ Ginsburg HJ. *From The Heart; Overcoming The Mental and Physical Trauma of Open Heart Surgery.* Denver: American Heart Association of Colorado; 1993.

CHAPTER 3--THE PRACTICAL WAY TO REVERSE BLOCKED ARTERIES!

♥ Hunninghake DB et al. The efficacy of intensive dietary therapy... *N Engl J Med.* 1993; 328(17):1213-19.

♥ Giovannucci E et al. A prospective study of dietary fat and risk of prostate cancer. *J Natl Cancer Inst.* 1993; 85(19):1571-79.

♥ Gould KL et al. Short term cholesterol lowering... *Circulation.* 1994; 89(4):1530-38.

♥ Morris DL et al. Serum carotenoids and coronary heart disease. *JAMA.* 1994; 272(18):1439-1441.

♥ White R and Frank E. Health effects and prevalence of vegetarianism. *West J Med.* 1994; 160:465.

CHAPTER 4--EATING RIGHT, THE PRACTICAL GUIDE

♥ Frahm A. *A Cancer Battle Plan.* Colorado Springs: Pinon Press; 1992.

♥ Debakey M. *The Living Heart Brand Name Shoppers Guide.* New York: Mastermedia Limited; 1993.

♥ Bellerson K. *The Complete and Up to Date Fat Book.* Garden City Park, NY: Avery Publishing Group; 1993.

♥ Moran V. *Get The Fat Out; 501 Simple Ways to Cut the Fat Out of Any Diet.* New York: Crown; 1994.

♥ Paino J, Messinger L. *The Tofu Book; The New American Cuisine.* Garden City Park, NY: Avery Publishing Group; 1991.

♥ Havala S, Clifford M. *Simple, Lowfat and Vegetarian; Unbelievably Easy Ways to Reduce the Fat in Your Meals.* Baltimore: Vegetarian Resource Group; 1994.

CHAPTER 5--THE FAT FREE EATERS'S GUIDE TO THE GROCERY STORE

♥ The New Food Label, Food and Drug Administration, 1993.

CHAPETR 6--EATING AWAY FROM HOME

♥ Warshaw H. *The Healthy Eater's Guide to Family and Chain Restaurants*. Wayzata, MN: Chronimed, 1993.

♥ Day B. *Fast Facts on Fast Food for Fast People*. Louisville, KY: An Apple A Day Publishing. 1995.

♥ Jacobson M, Fritschners. *The fast food Guide*, Rev & Updated. New Yor: Workman; 1991.

CHAPTER 7--WOMEN AND HEART DISEASE. THE WEAKER SEX?

♥ Gambrell RD. *The Menopause*. London: Blackwell Scientific Publications, Ltd; 1988; 247-261.

♥ Green LA, Ruffin MT. A closer examination of sex bias... *J Fam Pract*. 1994; 39:(4)331-6.

♥ Shaw LJ et al. Gender differences in the noninvasive evaluation of... *Ann Int Med*. 1994; 120:(7)559-66.

♥ Preuss HG. Nutrition and diseases of women: cardiovascular disorders. *J Am Coll Nutr*. 1993; 12(4):417-425.

♥ Peberdy MA, Ornato JP. Coronary artery disease in women. *Heart Dis Stroke*. 1992; 1(5):315-19.

♥ Nelson HD et al. Smoking, alcohol, and neuromuscular and physical function of older women. *JAMA*. 1994; 272(23):1825-31.

♥ Eaker E et al. Cardiovascular disease in women. *Circulation*. 1993; 88: 1999.

CHAPTER 8--SO WHAT'S STOPPING YOU?

♥ Moliterno DJ et al. Coronary vasoconstriction... *N Engl J Med*. 1994; 330(7):454-9.

♥ Kawachi I et al. Symptoms of anxiety and risk of coronary heart disease. *Circulation*. 1994; 90(5):2225-29.

♥ Carney RM et al. Major depressive disorder predicts cardiac events in patients with coronary artery disease. *Psychosom Med*. 1988; 50(6):627.

- ♥ Homes S. The social readjustment rating scale. *J of Psychosom Res.* 1967; 11:213-218.

- ♥ Eliot RS and Breo DL. *Is It Worth Dying For?.* New York: Bantam Books, 1986.

- ♥ Jiang T. *Mental Stress Testing.* Oxford, England. American Psychosomatic Society, Elsevier Science Ltd. Pergamon Imprint; 1994.

CHAPTER 9--MOVE YOUR BODY

- ♥ Blair SN et al. Physical fitness and all-cause mortality. *JAMA.* 1989; 262(17):2396-2401.

- ♥ Ainsworth BE. Compendium of physical activities: classification of energy costs of human activities. *Med Sci Sports Exerc.* 1993; 25(1)71-8.

- ♥ Anderson B. *Stretching.* Bolinas, CA: Shelter Publications, 1980.

- ♥ Franklin S. Exercise and cardiac complications. *The Physician and Sports Medicine.* 1994; (22)2: PAGE.

- ♥ Kelly G. Antihypertensive effects of aerobic exercise. *Am J Hypertens.* 1994; 7:115-119.

CHAPTER 10--KICK THE HABIT

- ♥ National Cancer Institute. How to help your patients stop smoking; 1994.

- ♥ Matzen. *Clinical Preventive Medicine.* Mosby: St. Louis, MO; 1993.

- ♥ Entire issue, The Journal of Family Practice, June 1992, vol. 34, no 6.

- ♥ Entire issue, Journal of the American Medical Association, Dec 11, 1991, vol. 266, no. 22.

- ♥ Glynn TJ. *How to Help Your Patients Stop Smoking.* Washington DC: National Institute of Health; 1990. NIH publication 90-3064.

CHAPTER 11--SHOULD I BE TAKING A SUPPLEMENT?

- National Institute of Health Consensus Conference, Optimal Calcium Intake. *JAMA*. 1994; 272(24)1942.

- McDougall J. *The McDougall Plan*. Clinton, NJ: New Win Publishing Inc.; 1983.

- Selhub J et al. Vitamin status and intake as primary determinants of homocysteinemia in an elderly population. *JAMA*. 1993; 270 (22):2693-98.

- Stampfer MJ et al. Vitamin E consumption and the risk of coronary artery disease in women. *N Engl J Med*. 1993; 328(20):1444-49.

- Schardt D. Phytochemicals: plants against cancer. *The Nutrition Action Health Letter*. 1994; 21(3):1.

- Morris DL et al. Serum carotenoids and coronary heart disease. *JAMA*. 1994; 272(18):1439-1441.

- Vita chart, Inc. 3611 Henry Hudson Parkway, #1d, Bronx, NY.

- Messina M, Messina V. *The Simple Soybean and Your Health*. Garden City Park, NY: Avery Publishing Group; 1994.

- Ulene A, Ulene V. *The Vitamin Strategy*. Berkeley: Ulysses Press; 1994.

- Somer E. *The Essential Guide to Vitamins and Minerals*. New York: Harper Collins; 1992.

CHAPTER 12--PHARMACEUTICAL

- Kessler D. Therapeutic class wars-drug promotion in a competitive marketplace. *N Engl Med*. 1994; 331(20):1350-1353.

- *The fifth report... high blood pressure*. Washington, DC: *National Institute of Health*; 1993. NIH publication no. 93-1088.

- *Second report on... high blood cholesterol in adults*. Washington, DC: *National Institute of Health*; 1993. NIH Publication no. 93-3095.

CHAPTER 13--A WORD ON CANCER PREVENTION

- ♥ Giovanucci E et al. A Prospective Study of Dietary Fat and Risk of Prostate Cancer. *J Natl Cancer Inst.* 1993; 85(19):1571-9.

- ♥ Howe GR et al. Dietary factors and risk of breast cancer... *J Natl Cancer Inst.* 1990; 82(7):561-69.

- ♥ Trock B et al. Dietary fiber, vegetables, and colon cancer... *J Natl Cancer Inst.* 1990; 82(8):650-61.

CHAPTER 14--DELIGHTFUL, DELICIOUS, DELECTIBLE RECIPES

- ♥ McDougall M. *The McDougall Health Supporting Cookbook.* New Win Publications Inc.: Berkeley; 1986.

- ♥ Hinman B, Snyder M. *Lean and Luscious and Meatless.* Rocklin, CA: Prima; 1992.

- ♥ Gilliard J, Kirkpatrick J. *Beyond Alfalfa Sprouts and Cheese; The Healthy Meatless Cookbook.* Wayzata, MN: Chronimed; 1993.

- ♥ Baird P. *Quick and Hearty Meatless Microwave Meals Everyone Will Enjoy.* New York: Henry Holt; 1991.

- ♥ Lakhani. *Indian Recipes for a Healthy Heart.* Los Angeles: Fahil Publishing; 1991 (this book is 75% vegetarian).

- ♥ Woodruff S. *The Secrets of Fat Free Baking.* Garden City Park, NY: Avery Publishing Group; 1994.

- ♥ Mateljan G. *Baking without Fat.* Irwindale, CA: Health Valley Foods; 1994.

- ♥ American Soybean Association, free recipes and information about soy products. 1-800-TALK-SOY.

- ♥ Vegetarian Resource Group, nonprofit group devoted to vegetarianism; publishes magazine and books. (410)-366-VEGE

CHAPTER 15-- CHOICES

- ♥ Ornish DM. Can lifestyle changes reverse coronary heart disease? *Lancet.* 1990; (336):129.

Order Form

Order additional copies of Make The Change For A Healthy Heart by mail, phone, fax or Email!

<u>Please send me:</u>   Total

_____ copies of Make The Change @ $14.95 $ _____

_____ I want to share the gift of good nutrition
        with friends! Send 3 copies @ 12.95 each $ 38.85

<u>Also from Fall River Press:</u>

_____ copies of Eating Expectantly, The Essential Eating
        Guide and Cookbook for Pregnancy @ $13.95 $ _____

<u>Shipping and Handling:</u>

$2.50 for 1st book; $1.00 for each additional book. $ _____

Colorado residents add sales tax--4.00% $ _____

Colorado Springs residents add sales tax--6.2% $ _____

<u>TOTAL ENCLOSED:</u> $ _____

Please enclose a check, money order or charge to your credit card:

Visa # _____ Expiration date: _____

Master Card # _____ Expiration date: _____

Name as it appears on on Card _____

Signature _____

<u>Ship to:</u>

Name: _____

Address: _____

Mail to:

Fall River Press

PO Box 62578 • Colorado Springs, CO 80962-2578

or

Phone your order to 1-800-284-6667

FAX your order using this form to 1-719-594-6124

Email your order to 75672.55@compuserve.com

Order Form

Order additional copies of Make The Change For A Healthy Heart by mail, phone, fax or Email!

Please send me: Total

_____ copies of Make The Change @ $14.95 $ _____

_____ I want to share the gift of good nutrition
with friends! Send 3 copies @ 12.95 each $ 38.85

Also from Fall River Press:

_____ copies of Eating Expectantly, The Essential Eating

Guide and Cookbook for Pregnancy @ $13.95 $ _____

Shipping and Handling:

$2.50 for 1st book; $1.00 for each additional book. $ _____

Colorado residents add sales tax--4.00% $ _____

Colorado Springs residents add sales tax--6.2% $ _____

TOTAL ENCLOSED: $ _____

Please enclose a check, money order or charge to your credit card:

Visa # _____Expiration date:_____

Master Card # _____Expiration date:_____

Name as it appears on on Card _____

Signature _____

Ship to:

Name: _____

Address: _____

Mail to:

Fall River Press

PO Box 62578 • Colorado Springs, CO 80962-2578

or

Phone your order to 1-800-284-6667

FAX your order using this form to 1-719-594-6124

Email your order to 75672.55@compuserve.com